THE MIGRAINE
HANDBOOK

THE MIGRAINE HANDBOOK

*The Definitive Guide to the Causes,
Symptoms and Treatments*

Jenny Lewis

with
The Migraine Action Association

VERMILION
LONDON

1 3 5 7 9 10 8 6 4 2

Text copyright © Jenny Lewis 1993, 1998

Jenny Lewis has asserted her right to be identified as the author of this work in accordance with the Copyright, Designs and Patents Act 1988.

First published in the United Kingdom in 1993 by Vermilion

This edition published in the United Kingdom in 1998 by Vermilion
an imprint of Ebury Press
Random House
20 Vauxhall Bridge Road
London SW1V 2SA

Random House Australia (Pty) Limited
20 Alfred Street, Milsons Point, Sydney,
New South Wales 2061, Australia

Random House New Zealand Limited
18 Poland Road, Glenfield,
Auckland 10, New Zealand

Random House South Africa (Pty) Limited
Endulini, 5A Jubilee Road,
Parktown 2192, South Africa

Random House UK Limited Reg. No. 954009
A CIP catalogue record for this book is available from the British Library

ISBN: 0 09 181666 1
Printed and bound by Mackays of Chatham plc

Contents

Foreword

This book needed to be written – it was a book looking for an author. When Jenny Lewis agreed to become the editor of our newsletter and demonstrated her talent, energy, compassion and humour, it became obvious that here was the right person for the job.

Migraine sufferers do not always know a great deal about their migraine, they need to learn about their enemy. *The Migraine Handbook* has been written to help them do that; it is packed with information to help sufferers control their attacks and to encourage and guide them through the maze of contradictions and frustrations that can bedevil migraineurs. By talking to a large number of Migraine Action Association members who had volunteered to help, Jenny collected vivid descriptions of what living with migraine meant to each one. These moving first-hand accounts illustrate the huge diversity of migraine and its consequences. They should go a long way towards promoting a greater understanding of migraine; they are a unique feature of this book.

For many people, the biggest benefit to be gained from *The Migraine Handbook* is the knowledge that they are not alone; the strange symptoms and feelings they experience are not unique; they are not going crazy, and thousands of other people understand. *The Migraine Handbook* is so full of good advice. Read it, and read it again. Keep it by you to consult and to remind you of things you can try. It could be a valuable weapon in your campaign against migraine and its miseries. We have won some battles but we haven't won the war yet – fight on!

Jo Liddell
Director, British Migraine Association (now known as the
Migraine Action Association) 1981 – 1996

Introduction

Why this book?

There are many ways of looking at migraine. The scientist will ponder over your blood vessels and body chemicals, the psychologist will wonder about your state of mind, the allergist will look at your diet, the bone people will be concerned with your bones and the acupuncturist will do clever things with needles. In the meantime you, the patient, will be clutching your head, throwing up into the nearest receptacle and wondering what you've done to deserve this.

Many excellent medical books have been written on the subject of migraine, several of which are quoted and referred to in this one. When trying to combat any illness, it is useful to have some knowledge of the medical background. So I have included descriptions of symptoms, different types of migraines and some of the treatments currently available, as well as hints, tips and information gathered from sufferers themselves. But this book is written by a migraine sufferer on behalf of the Migraine Action Association and as such is primarily concerned with what it *feels* like to have migraine. There are over forty personal accounts published here and although names have been changed, every story is a true one. Both the Migraine Action Association and I would like to thank everybody who agreed to be interviewed and have their stories published here.

If you suffer from migraine, I hope that you will read this book and never again feel embarrassed, ashamed, odd, malingering or insane. Because your neighbour two doors down can go off to work with a migraine, it doesn't mean that you can. For some people a migraine is a headache that they can work through. For others it is an illness that affects the whole body and sends them to bed for several hours or even days. Migraine can claim a large chunk of the patient's life.

If you are the husband, wife, child or parent of a migraine sufferer you probably know by now how it is for us. And we know how it is for you. How many husbands come home evening after evening, tired and hungry, to find their dinner still in the freezer and their wife shut away in the bedroom? How many times have you, the partner, had to say: 'I'm sorry, I've had to come on my own because my wife/husband has another migraine.' Do you feel ridiculous? You are not alone. What about the children? Do they still look forward to promised outings or do they pull the face that says: 'Maybe it will happen and then again maybe it won't.'

How many wives have stood by helplessly while their husbands suffer the excruciating agony of a cluster headache night after night. And how many, dependent on their husband's earnings, fear that this bout of clusters or migraines will cost them their jobs and their lifestyles.

The Migraine Action Association believes that there is some hope for every single sufferer somewhere out there. You may not be able to cure the migraine but you should be able to find a therapy which lessens either the severity or the frequency of attacks – or both. It's a question of looking – not easy but worth the effort especially if your migraines are frequent, severe and disruptive. Don't give up. It's not hopeless. Most people can find something that helps them manage their migraines.

I hope it will not be only the general public who read this book. Although no medical breakthroughs are offered here, sufferers are presenting their symptoms and offering a glimpse into their lives. It should help doctors to understand beyond the headaches, the nausea and the flashing lights. Many patients are helped just by being diagnosed. Giving the pain a name can bring enormous relief when the diagnosis does not spell 'fatal illness'. Every patient is helped by an understanding doctor. Knowing what goes on at home can help you to prescribe. We know you can't cure us, so we can't accuse you of failing us in that. But you let us down when you don't give our illness the importance it deserves: migraine may not kill us, but it often destroys our lives.

Do you get migraines?

Migraines are often confused with sinus or other types of headache. So perhaps the first step is to find out if what you suffer from is migraine. Here's a quick checklist.

When you have a headache, do you:

- Sometimes 'know' it's coming before it hurts?
- Feel a throbbing deep in your head?
- Feel the pain in one side of your head?
- Get queasy and perhaps vomit when your head is painful?
- Cry with pain or think you are going mad?
- Find that your eyes go funny – that you see flashes or zigzags? Or do things look dark or 'patterned' or strange?

- Look so pale and drawn that your family or friends comment on how ill you look?
- Dislike noise or light?
- Dislike to be touched?
- Want to get away from the family when normally if you're unwell you like to be comforted?
- Feel that your sense of smell is different?
- Notice that the pain gets worse if you move?
- Get tingling in your limbs?
- Find it usually lasts between four hours and three days?

A 'Yes' to one or more of these questions means that you may well suffer from migraines. If you were car-sick a lot as a child this can be a pointer as well; and although there is no hard scientific evidence to prove that migraine is genetically inherited, the illness does seem to run in families. According to Dr J. N. Blau in *Understanding Headaches and Migraines*, published by the Consumers' Association and Hodder and Stoughton, migraine sufferers have about a 60 per cent chance of having a relative who also has migraines.

Migraine is a benign recurring headache that is not a symptom of anything more serious. The patient is symptom-free between the attacks. It used to be thought that migraine started at puberty and ended at the menopause for women and in their fifties for men. Now it seems that it can start in childhood and go on well into the - seventies – some people are stuck with the affliction to their dying day. Most sufferers have their first attack before the age of twenty, and around one in eight before they are ten years old. A first attack of migraine after the age of fifty has been known, but it is rare.

There is a myth that migraine sufferers tend to be more intelligent than their fellow humans but there is no scientific evidence to support this comforting theory. It could have arisen because the sufferers who ask their doctors for help tend to come from the professional and managerial classes, but this may well have more to do with confidence than with intelligence! So anyone can suffer from it, though roughly three times as many women as men are affected.

Different types of migraine

The International Headache Society, which is a multi-national society of neurologists, has devised a system for classifying headaches and migraines. This is an attempt to unify, on a worldwide basis, what we mean when we give a head pain a name.

Migraine without aura

If you go anywhere in the world and say you suffer from 'migraine without aura' (old name: common migraine), the doctor will know that you have headaches that last between four and seventy-two hours. They are likely to be of the pulsating kind, one-sided and moderate to severe in intensity, and they will have at least two of these attributes. The headaches will also include at least one of these symptoms: nausea and/or vomiting, and sensitivity to light and/or sound. The pain gets worse as you move around. These migraines were known as 'common' because many more people suffer from them than other types of migraine. They can greatly affect sufferers' lives. A full description of this type of migraine and personal accounts of sufferers appears in Chapter 1.

Migraine with aura

Formerly known as classical migraine, this includes the neurological symptoms known as an aura, which is described fully in Chapter 2. The aura normally lasts about half an hour and is followed by headache, nausea and sensitivity to light and/or sound. There may be a gap between the aura ending and the headache starting. Sometimes people only suffer the aura sensation and no headache.

Tension-type headaches

Previously known as tension headaches, these can last from half an hour to one week. They have a pressing or tightening quality. The pain may be only mild, no more than discomfort, and have more to do with the pressing/tightening sensation which affects both sides of the head. Physical movement makes no difference. Patients can experience mild nausea but there is no vomiting and sensitivity to light or sound is unlikely.

Migraine Without Aura

Warning signs

Many migraine sufferers get warning of an impending attack. Since migraine is very painful and debilitating you would expect warning signs to come in the shape of gloom and malaise. It can happen this way, but many sufferers experience quite the opposite – an amazing up-swing in mood and energy. For some people the very earliest inkling of an attack can be that they feel unusually happy, energetic and alive. One patient described it as a sensation of euphoria, when she feels she's re-entered her life as an eighteen-year-old (she's sixty-five!). Is this yet another of life's little ironies, or is there a scientific explanation? Medically speaking, it is thought that these sensations stem from a temporary chemical imbalance in the area of the brain which is responsible for our emotions. The hypothalamus controls the secretions of several hormones, and it may be that an alteration here sets the scene for an attack.

Although these feelings of elation are not uncommon, other sufferers receive quite different signals. They will feel weak, run down and generally off-colour. They may yawn a lot, experience diarrhoea or constipation, feel tense, depressed and irritable and be extremely sensitive to light, sound or smell. Hunger and thirst are two early warning symptoms worth a special mention, because every now and again you may be able to abort a migraine by doing what comes naturally – giving in to them. If you feel thirsty – drink. Three glasses of not too cold water will flush out the kidneys and may prevent an attack. If you feel hungry – eat. No jam doughnuts – in fact avoid all sugary food – but carbohydrates and protein will keep the blood sugar at the right level and provide the body with the right ammunition to help fight off an attack. Your diet you can worry about later.

Symptoms

The two main symptoms of migraine without aura are headache and nausea.

Headache

The headache is usually a violent throbbing pain – often in one temple. But although it may start on one side of the head it often spreads to more or the rest of the head as it develops. Some patients find that their migraine starts on the same side of the head each time, while with others it changes from attack to attack. The throbbing usually gives way to a steady aching. Patients can often feel the tenderness on the affected part of the head just by touching it.

Moving the head, coughing, sneezing or vomiting usually aggravates the pain, bringing about the throbbing sensation. So stillness and rest are definitely advocated. Some people find that pressing the affected part of the head into a pillow helps. A hot water bottle placed on the site of the pain can provide a degree of relief for some patients, while others find that an ice pack has a beneficial effect. (A packet of frozen vegetables makes a good ice pack!)

Some people's migraines are violently painful and totally incapacitating, while other sufferers are only slightly aware of its existence. The intense pain is not necessarily felt all through the attack. There is a little light relief when the pain lessens before rising to a crescendo again.

Nausea

The nausea that almost always accompanies this type of migraine can be slight, or it can be even more uncomfortable than the headache itself. Many patients are not able to eat during an attack. The smell of food, apart from anything else, can make the nausea worse.

Gastric symptoms

Hiccuping, belching, retching and vomiting are also part and parcel of some attacks. Luckier people can be sick and end their attack at that point, but with most patients the vomiting aggravates the issue by making the headache even more painful. Each time the person vomits, the contents of the stomach are depleted until the sufferer is bringing up nothing but bile, followed by heaving and retching. Many people also experience stomach ache, which may be colicky.

Red and white migraines

Sufferers' faces often change colour. Some people have what are known as 'red migraines'. These patients go dusky and flushed in the face and they are usually people who tend to blush or go red with anger. 'White migraines' are more common: the sufferer goes very pale and drawn and looks ill, with heavily ringed, sunken eyes. Some people's eyes become bloodshot and itchy and there may be a burning sensation.

Vision

Sensitivity to light (photophobia) is an extremely common feature of this type of migraine and sufferers can be so severely affected that they have to remain in a darkened room with their eyes covered. In order to try and understand photophobia, think what it is like to go from a very dark room into bright sunlight without wearing sunglasses. That immediate discomfort is similar to what is felt by a light-sensitive migraine sufferer.

Smell

Although it has been known for some time that the eyes are affected in migraine attacks, what hasn't been so well documented is the effect on the nasal passages. This has led to many migraine patients being erroneously treated for sinus problems. Stuffiness of the nose can be experienced, and there may be heavy catarrh and a sharp, knife-like pain when breathing. Some patients can press the outside of their nose and actually feel the tenderness there. Patients can also be very sensitive to smell, a condition known as osmophobia. One sufferer freaked out when her daughter applied a tiny drop of perfume as far away as the next bedroom. Another recalled that, when her husband added a clove of garlic to the stew he was cooking in the kitchen, she picked up the smell as she was lying in her bedroom and consequently threw up.

Intolerance of noise

Phonophobia – an intolerance to noise – is very common during attacks. In the same way as the person affected by osmophobia is hypersensitive to smells, the phonophobic has a highly increased awareness of sounds. A clock which ticks quietly and unnoticed in the room at other times can be as disturbing as hammering during an attack. Many sufferers say that they cannot tolerate the sound of footsteps even on a carpeted floor and for this reason do not want anyone to come into the room. Most migraine sufferers like to be left alone, and when you understand that the minutest of sounds, smells and light can aggravate the situation you can see why. A visitor sitting themselves down on the bed, even very gently, can turn the sufferer's ache into a throb!

Other symptoms

An increase in fluid retention is experienced by some patients, who say that they swell up during an attack. Frequent urination is also common. Dizziness and a feeling of light-headedness are two other well-known symptoms.

After the attack

A migraine attack can end with the sufferer dropping off to sleep sometimes waking up feeling very refreshed and even euphoric. Or the attack can just gradually disappear. More often than not sufferers are left feeling very weak, washed-out and debilitated, and this can last for a day or two.

Treatment

There are a variety of painkillers and other kinds of drugs on the market that alleviate or lessen the severity of attacks. Many patients find that a painkiller like aspirin or paracetamol is sufficient, particularly if taken with an anti-sickness pill like Stemetil (prochloperazine). But some patients find that painkillers don't do much good. This may be because by the time they come to take drug treatment the stomach has 'shut down' and very little is being absorbed. This condition is known as gastric stasis. The drug given in this situation is Maxolon (metoclopramide) which makes the stomach empty faster so that the drugs pass into the small intestine and are absorbed more easily. Maxolon is also an anti-sickness drug. The idea is to take Maxolon about ten to fifteen minutes before the preferred painkiller. There is a drug available on prescription which combines paracetamol and Maxolon and this is Paramax. There is also one that contains aspirin and Maxolon called Migravess. The latter is effervescent. Another prescription drug used in this way is Motilium (domperidone). This remedy does not cause drowsiness.

Some stronger over-the-counter painkillers contain a small amount of codeine in addition to aspirin or paracetamol as well as an antihistamine. This combination seems to be particularly helpful to migraine sufferers. Two of these remedies are Migraleve and Syndol.

Further details of some of the drugs used in the treatment of migraine appear in Chapter 11.

So much for symptoms and treatment. In the next four stories sufferers not only describe their symptoms but, in many ways more importantly, they tell you how migraine has affected their lives.

Anna

I am now sixteen years old, but I was fourteen when I first started suffering from migraine. I had no idea what it was that made me ill until I had been having migraine for eighteen months. They were diagnosed as common migraine. I got them as often as once a week. At first I thought my attacks were hangovers or a violent allergy to the food I ate, as I always got them after a Friday or Saturday night. But I knew it had to be something different as I was often ill for a whole day and I never recovered until I had had a good night's sleep.

My symptoms included an unbelievably painful headache over my left eye. It was the piercing sort and usually the rest of my head ached as well. Very soon afterwards I would be nauseous as if I was on the verge of vomiting. This lasted for several hours. I would become so weak I would have to lie down and eventually I would vomit. I would keep vomiting until I was dehydrated. Because of this I became quite thin.

I was always annoyed with myself for being this way as I had no understanding of what it was. I found that Paracetamol or aspirin didn't help and this baffled me all the more.

My migraine attacks always seemed to come at the wrong time – when I was staying with someone or if I was out with friends. I felt very guilty as I couldn't pretend I was all right like you can with a normal headache. I always had to be taken home, and when I got there my mother would sigh and say: 'You're not ill again are you?'

I missed out on a lot of things and I let a lot of people down. The attacks were so frequent that my friends and family could recognize them even before I could, as they said I always went pale and didn't speak if I was about to have an attack.

Eighteen months later I decided that this wasn't normal and couldn't be an allergy to food or drink as my attacks followed no particular pattern. I went to my doctor and he told me I suffered from migraines. We tried all sorts of medication: Migraleve and Paramax tablets. These didn't work for me so now I take Sanomigran every day, which although they make me very drowsy, work extremely well.

After Anna was diagnosed as a migraine sufferer, her mother contacted the Migraine Action Association and was sent information on the illness. This not only helped her mother understand what Anna was going through, but Anna herself was able to explain the nature of the illness to her friends. Two years later I contacted Anna to see how things were going. She is still on Sanomigran every day, and although she still gets migraines they are much more manageable. She still gets a headache, but it is not as bad as before and she very rarely vomits. In addition, the frequency of attacks is down to roughly one a month, usually appearing a week after her period. Anna is able to continue with her work and social life very much as normal. One of the gripes about Sanomigran is that it tends to make you put on weight. Anna says that she does have to watch her diet, but she is not sure whether this is due to Sanomigran or the fact that she has stopped vomiting during attacks!

Cynthia

When I was young I had what were then called bilious attacks but which I now know was migraine. Then I didn't have it during my teens. I had one on my wedding day. On the way down to Cornwall we had to keep stopping the car as I was getting sick. Directly we got to the hotel I said: 'I'm going to bed.' I didn't want any dinner. So my poor husband wasn't given any either. I didn't have any more migraines until my son was six months old.

They were diagnosed as common migraines. I get a very bad headache. I get nauseous and I'm very often sick – sometimes so much so that the doctor has to come in to give me something to stop it. I had a hysterectomy when I was forty-one. Ten years later, my husband died and the migraines really got going after that. He had cancer and I nursed him at home for nine months. The funny thing is that I can only remember having one migraine attack during all that time.

After he died I had a lot of adjusting to do. I didn't know about any-thing. I was very dependent on him. I'd never worked throughout our marriage. Whatever he said went and he made all the decisions on how the money was spent. I think a lot of women of my generation were like that. I'd never signed a cheque. After he died I pushed myself to my limits. I felt somehow that I had to justify my existence. At one time I had five students living in my home and I was sleeping downstairs. That takes some doing! I was getting migraines then but they weren't that bad.

I fell down in the street and broke my knee-cap. It was traumatic. Then I broke my ankle and after that I fell down in the bedroom and broke my leg. The doctor said that all these accidents were a shock to the system. My migraines started to come very frequently – two or three times a week. I began to feel I just could not cope any longer. I became very depressed. I kept feeling that there was something wrong with me and I was seeing different specialists. One diagnosed this terrible feel-ing I had as stomach migraine. I now know I was suffering from chronic anxiety. I gradually went into a clinical depression. Eventually I had a nervous breakdown.

I got psychiatric help. The worst time was the several weeks when I was in the deep depression. I was allowed to stay at home during those weeks because a man I had met after my husband died offered to stay with me and help me through. I was in a deep pit. I was suicidal some of the time. I wasn't interested in anything. I hardly ate. I lost a lot of weight. It's the most terrible form of suffering I can describe, and unfortunately people have no idea. They feel you should pull yourself together. But that's the very thing you can't do. While I was in the pit I didn't have a single migraine. But as I started to climb out of it – they came back.

They aren't as bad now, however. I get them once or twice a week, but I take Cafergot at the start of an attack and it very often aborts it. I can carry on as normal.

My mother used to get migraines. I can see her now, lying in bed all day never moving, poor soul I had no comprehension then of how she suffered.

Diana

It can be any time. There's no pattern. I can't tolerate the light but I don't get any visual disturbances. It usually starts in the morning. I sort of feel tired and then I feel as if I've got a really heavy band around my head. I feel very sick but I'm not often actually sick. I go and lie down and it will last all day. The band gets tighter but I also get a headache. It's from the top of the bridge of the nose really. It's a throbbing, sick headache at the front of the head.

I lie in bed in the dark. I've got relaxation tapes or very soothing music. I can't listen to the radio because I can't stand the noise. I can't eat or drink.

I think my migraines are stress related. I have elderly parents whom I have to look after, they don't speak to each other so it's very complicated. I don't live with them, but when I come back – I don't know if it is a self-fulfilling prophecy – that's when I usually get the migraines. I started having them when I was twenty-six. Before then I wasn't the headache type. I'm forty-one now.

I am the only child of my adoptive parents. They were OK when I was a child, but I was always aware that there was something the matter with the relationship. It wasn't a very cohesive family at all and now my parents have little contact with one another. I look after them. I do everything really. They refuse to have any help in the house. I do all the cleaning, cooking, shopping and so on. Then if you talk to one the other one sulks. It's exhausting.

Originally I was prescribed Migril, which is what I have taken all the time since. I take the tablets at the start of the attack. I don't know whether they help or not, because I don't know how bad the migraines would be if I didn't take them – I don't dare not take them. I take one to start with, and then if it's fairly bad I take another one in the afternoon.

But I don't take more than six in a week. But that's what I take roughly twice a month.

Migraine sufferers commonly forget about the illness between attacks, and as a result they often have difficulty in recalling their symptoms even days after an attack. Indeed, it is not unusual for sufferers to convince themselves that they are never going to get another attack. Maybe it is because so many patients feel so well between attacks that they can't believe they are going to have another one. Whatever the reason, Louise feels that her mother has taken this syndrome too far.

Louise

My mother was a migraine sufferer. She's seventy-nine and I asked her the other day about her migraine and she said she's never had it. Now I think that's really weird. I don't know if she's got senile dementia or whether Mother Nature has been wonderfully kind and obliterated it completely from her memory, but I have a childhood memory of her walking around with one of my dad's ties tied round her head like a Mohican, banging her head on the living room wall – and she's forgotten it. I can't believe it. She used to walk around with squinty eyes. The pain must have been really bad. But she can't remember having a headache. Her memory seems to be OK in every other respect. She forgets the odd thing, but I think I forget more things than she does.

Mine started three months before I got married. I was on holiday when I had this humdinger of a headache and I thought 'Oh my God'. That was the very first one. I didn't have them when I was pregnant, but quite soon after the babies were born I was back on the old treadmill. When I was breast-feeding my next door neighbour had to take my baby away from me and bring her back every four hours to be fed. How I had any milk for her was a mystery, because I wasn't eating or drinking. I loved breast-feeding. I felt so guilty that I couldn't look after my kid. I thought: 'I've just got to do this.' I was probably weeping all over her at the time. I just felt awful that I had to ask other people to help me. I was getting a couple of migraines a week at that stage.

In a typical attack I wake up with one and I don't know how long it is since it started. If I get three paracetamol down at the right stage I'm fine. But if it's in full swing by then I'm like it for two or three days on end. I had it for five days once last year. I'd be sick all the time. I have to lie in bed like a mummy – not moving a muscle. Even talking to my kids makes me sick. All I want is hot water bottles. I find the heat helps. I've tried cold, but it's agony. I lie with my face into the pillow and the hot water bottle. It's a wonder I haven't got a red, blotchy, scarred face now lying like this over the years. I usually have to wear bed socks and a cardigan because I'm cold. I just drink filtered water. I have a jug of water and a bucket by my side and I just want to be left alone.

On good days I'm chasing around trying to catch up because I'm in bed so much. I can take on the world when I'm feeling well. I get a sense of euphoria.

My two kids have had to grow up very quickly and become independent. Everybody in the family suffers – not just me. When we first got married my husband used to feel a prisoner in his own house. He was aware that I was upstairs being ill and didn't want anyone there. He felt guilty about going out. He spent weekends on his own. When the kids came along it was: 'Don't make a noise, Mummy's in bed.' 'Don't bang your football up against the wall.' They've had to suffer as well. Trips were cancelled and so on. My husband now goes to dinner parties and other social events on his own. He gets back late from work and then he comes upstairs and massages my neck. He empties my sick bucket. His stomach is rumbling like mad. He's come all the way from London and it's nine o'clock at night and there's no food in the oven or anywhere near the table and he has to dive into the freezer and defrost something. He doesn't sit down until about half past ten. I mean, he moans occasionally but on the whole he's very good. He feels angry, frustrated and helpless.

I've been to several hospitals and migraine clinics, but to no avail. I've had faith healing, acupuncture, different diets, I've had my hair tested and I've drunk all sorts of weird concoctions. I went to a herbalist. She said I should drink my own urine every morning. I couldn't. I just couldn't. I thought: 'I've got wonderful friends – I don't want to lose them.'

I'm on Sanomigran and I've put on so much weight – over a stone. I'm walking around as if I'm pregnant. I've got this tummy in front of me. I feel lethargic with it. I can't wear any of my size 10 clothes any more. But I can't do much strenuous exercise to take it off because it makes me feel ill. The drug has helped me, but I'm fighting a losing battle with the flab.

I did a massage course four years ago because I thought it would be very therapeutic for me. It has been wonderful. It really helps me. I do it from home, using essential oils. As soon as I put my hands on someone I relax. My heart slows down. But I did it primarily because I suffer from migraines.

2

Migraine With Aura

Symptoms

Aura

The onset of this type of attack is the aura which can comprise a number of symptoms. As you read the stories in this chapter you will see that patients suffer from a variety of quite scary experiences, though virtually all of them are visual disturbances of one kind or another. It is not unusual for someone who has a classical migraine attack for the first time to feel that they are going blind or sometimes even mad. Sufferers commonly see a spot in front of the eye which gradually increases in size until it covers nearly the whole field of vision. This blind spot is known as a scotoma. For others the vision will blur, or they may see flashing lights, zigzags or a Catherine wheel in front of their eyes. These disturbances are thought to be caused by the narrowing of blood vessels feeding the brain, which means that less blood is getting to the brain. Other symptoms caused by this restricted blood flow are a feeling of numbness, usually starting in one side of the face or in one arm, which may be followed by weakness in the same part of the body. Very rarely, people can lose consciousness and suffer blackouts (see Joelle's story on p. 16).

When the headache comes on it will usually be on the side of the body that hasn't been affected by weakness or numbness. Patients will often be confused, unable to collect their thoughts or to speak coherently. They may feel dizzy and not be able to tolerate light or any sounds or smells.

Sometimes during the aura sufferers experience an apparent change in the objects around them. The teapot, for instance, may look larger or smaller than usual. It may seem further away, or appear to be tilted when it is standing quite straight. Sufferers may see things that are not there, or they may feel themselves to have grown larger or smaller. Lewis Carroll, the author of *Alice in Wonderland*, suffered from migraine. It was thought at one time that some of Alice's experiences were a re-enactment of his own migraines, but apparently he only started suffering from this complaint after he had written the book. Maybe, along with his very considerable imagination and writing talents, he had the gift of premonition!

It is not known how many people suffer from mild hallucinations and see things that aren't there or experience objects changing in size or shape. Sadly, very few people admit to it for fear of being thought peculiar or – worse – mentally ill. But when you look at the aura from a scientific standpoint and realize that all these effects are simply a consequence of restricted blood flow to the brain, it doesn't seem very odd at all. Some people suffer a mild constriction of the blood vessels while others have to put up with a more severe one – hence the extremes of experience.

Headache and associated symptoms

The aura can last from about twenty minutes to one hour and is usually, but not always, followed by a severe headache. This can start on one side of the head and then become more generalized, and is often accompanied by nausea, vomiting and diarrhoea. As in migraine without aura, patients suffering from this type of migraine can be extremely sensitive to light, sound and smell. Tenderness in the head or neck either during or after an attack is common.

Treatment

Over the years migraine sufferers have tried all manner of different treatments involving both drug-based and non-drug therapies. As you read the stories in this book you will see that what works for one person may be useless for somebody else. Some people will find a solution to their migraines quite easily in their doctor's surgery or through a specialist. Others will stumble across a non-drug therapy which suits them. But some will have exhausted medical expertise and knocked on the doors of virtually all the alternative therapists to no avail. This is because migraine has so many different causes that it is different for each individual.

David, in this next story, is pinning his hopes on feverfew – a herb which has helped a great many migraine sufferers. Chapter 13 discusses the alternative therapies that have helped sufferers. Drug therapy has helped many patients manage their migraines. But there are possible side-effects, so a balancing act has to be worked out. Obviously, the benefits must considerably outweigh the possible unwanted side-effects for the drug to be worth taking. But bear in mind that many of the drugs used in migraine are highly effective and have changed the lives of severe sufferers. If the pills the GP gives you don't work, don't throw them away and give up. Go back and tell your doctor. Give him a chance to try something else. If he cannot find a solution for you, ask your GP to refer you to a neurologist or a migraine clinic. Chapter 10 discusses this part of migraine management more fully. If you want a good idea of what an aura is like, read David's story:

David

It will happen in one of two ways. I'll have a small dot in the middle which will then expand and go into the letter C and this will go into either one corner of my vision or the other. Or I'll suddenly be aware of a blank space to one side of my vision which will do the same thing eventually. At this point I see criss-cross lines and dots in front of my eyes.

Although I can't focus properly I don't lose my vision completely because I can see around the dot, and when the C shape is there I can see in the middle. I've never suffered from sickness, but I sometimes get slight nausea.

The aura can last anything up to half an hour. This can be followed by a headache, but not always. Sometimes I just feel stupid. I get muddled and can't concentrate my thoughts. I know what I want to say but the words won't come out properly. I also get numbness. This can come completely on its own – nothing to do with the aura or anything else. The numbness will start on one side and then run across and then just disappear. A migraine may come on afterwards.

My migraines have never really affected my job or my social life in the past. They weren't that frequent. Latterly, in the last three years, I started getting ten a month which is rather different. A couple of months ago I started taking feverfew. I got four attacks last month and so far, a fortnight into this month, I haven't had any. So here's hoping!

It is surprising how many migraine sufferers are both able and enthusiastic at sport. Thirteen-year-old Jane is exceptionally supple and talented in this way, to the extent that she was told by a professional gymnast that if she trained she could become professional herself. Although Jane did not want to take it quite that seriously she is still very committed to sports in general and gymnastics in particular.

Jane

My vision becomes very blurred. It's like I've got a film in front of my eyes. There are squirls of light. This happens for about half an hour and then the headache comes on. Sometimes if I take an aspirin at this point I don't get a headache, but other times it makes no difference. I get very hot and my arm and legs feel really tired. The headache is not just in the forehead – it's everywhere. It's like I've got a headache in my arms and legs. I can't bear to hear sounds – footsteps or anything like that. I can feel them vibrate. I can hear the footsteps in my arms. I feel very sick. I don't like people talking to me because it sounds too loud. If I try to speak I get sick. I can't drink anything – not even water. It lasts for about two or three hours and then I go to sleep.

I try not to give in to them. The other day I had the aura in the morning. I took a Disprin and it went away. I went to school. Me and my friend were going to the gym club in the evening. As I said goodbye to my mum I had the funny eyes. I had the squirls and a vague headache. I tried to ignore it. When I started in the gym I got the headache and I became very hot. I didn't do the bar work because I was worried. I tried to do a headstand but my head felt really heavy and I couldn't push up to the headstand because my arms were hurting. I asked the lady if I could sit down because I had a migraine, and she was very nice and said I could.

I went to the loo and was sick twice. I washed my face and went out again. A little girl I had been doing gym with looked at me and said: 'Ugh! Your face is green – green!' I was dreading the car journey home. Car journeys are really bad. I'm frightened of being sick. It's so embarrassing. When my friend said it was time to go home I went to the loo and made myself sick. I thought if I was sick then I would be all right on the way home. Everyone was really quiet in the car because I think they got the message that I really didn't want to speak. I feel guilty when that happens. I kept swallowing so that the sick wouldn't come. Every time I swallowed it came and went. My head was throbbing but the funny eyes had gone and I could see properly. When I got home I went straight to bed.

Jane, whose migraines started when she was about ten, suffers them about every two months.

Joelle, who also suffers from classical migraines, has a very different story to tell. Now eighty-one, she has been a sufferer for sixty years. Joelle's migraines are so unusual that her specialist told her he had only read of one other case like hers and that was in Australia.

Joelle
There's no pattern to my migraines. One month I might have six, the next, two or three. Either way, I never have an attack without an aura.

It starts with impaired vision. If I was to look at your face I would suddenly realize that I couldn't see the whole of it. I'd see three-quarters. All of a sudden a very tiny spot of light emerges and it gets bigger and bigger. Then it zigzags all the way round until it covers practically my whole field of vision. It gets bigger and bigger until it is nearly a circle. It never achieves a complete circle. Then it gradually goes back the same way as it came and gets weaker and weaker.

I used to get a very severe headache following this, but nowadays the pain is not so bad and sometimes I don't get a headache at all. On twelve occasions during my sixty years of migraine I have blacked out. Once I blacked out in Marks and Spencer's and woke up in hospital'!

My migraines have affected me in that I've always got them at the back of my mind. Even on my wedding day I made sure I had some Cafergot in the pocket of my outfit. They've tried various tablets on me but I'm one of these people who are allergic to pills so nowadays I more or less have to grin and bear it.

Although they are such rare occurrences, I'm terrified of the blackouts. When I was working I was in charge of telephonists. If I got a warning I would tell the girls I had a migraine coming and would retire to the rest room. I was frightened of blacking out in front of them. I did once and I lost my job through it. I was given some silly excuses for being given notice. I felt very cut up about it. A long time afterwards I realized that the girls got so worried about me passing out that they didn't like me working there.

When I get an aura I turn everything off and sit very comfortably away from anything I could crash into should I pass out. I look at the clock to see the time and I can tell then that it will be over in about twenty minutes and I can feel safe again. But it doesn't always work out that way. Two years ago I passed out in the corridor. I think I must have been on my way to the kitchen to turn off the gas – I was cooking something. Anyway, when I came round I was on the floor caught between the two doorways and I couldn't get out of the position I was in. I must have been on the floor for about two hours before I could get to my feet. My neighbour called an ambulance. I suffered a triple fracture of the collar bone.

If I get the aura and I'm outside it takes me all my time not to panic. I find myself saying: 'Please God, let me get home safely.' Apart from any injury, I can't bear to make an exhibition of myself. I won't get on a bus or anything until it is over in case I pass out. If there is anywhere I can sit down, I do that until it is over. Suppose, for instance, the aura starts in church, I'll come out. If I wasn't able to get out I should never want to go back there again. It gets me to that extent. If I passed out I'd feel I'd made an exhibition of myself. I know it's silly. People tell me not to worry, but I do. I started life as a rather quiet, nervous person. I had eight years as a boarder in a convent and I came out very well aware of what I must and mustn't do. I've always been a tense person. I think it's *got something to do with it. But that's not going to change. Not now. Not with this following me around.*

Early diagnosis for a sufferer of migraine with aura is a boon. Not only are they reassured that they do not have a brain tumour or a serious eye problem, but they are relieved to find that they are not going 'funny' in any way!

Susan
The first time I thought I was going blind. I was really quite frightened. It was just before my twenty-first birthday. I was at work, just talking to a colleague, and I looked at her and saw the lights and she was disappearing. I could only see half of her. I thought: 'I can't see!' I went home terrified and the doctor came the next morning. He diagnosed it as migraine immediately. I was lucky. At least I knew what it was and knew there wasn't anything wrong with my sight.

That was thirty-two years ago. I started by getting the classical ones. Things would change colour. I would get the flashing lights and the headache would come on within half an hour once they had stopped. When I was on ergotamine I would get pins and needles in my face. I went through one stage when I couldn't speak properly. It was as if the migraine was in my mouth and I was talking rubbish.

When I was about thirty-five they changed to common migraines. I get them every fortnight to three weeks now, and they last about three days each time. I have pain down my right shoulder and I feel the tension coming. Then it is into my neck and behind my right eye and the whole right-hand side of my head. I start to feel sick and I keep on yawning. I feel very tired and I can't keep awake and then the pain gets worse.

I live in Northants, and work in London, so it's a long journey every day. When I feel an attack coming on I start to worry how I'm going to get home. I get very tense and it makes things worse. They're very good at work. But the worst thing is planning what you can do. I can't make arrangements because I don't know when the migraines are going to come. I hate having so much time off work. You have to catch up when you get back. Very often people think it's just another headache. They don't realize just how ill you feel. It's not the sort of pain you can work through.

I've lain across bus seats and thought: 'I wish they'd arrest me and put me in prison, because I can't do this journey home.' I did almost go into a police station once and ask to be put up for the night because I felt so awful. But I pulled myself together and got on a bus and lay across the back seat. The bus conductor didn't seem to mind. You wouldn't dream of doing that in the normal course of events. But when you've got a migraine you feel taken over by something else completely.

It is not unusual for sufferers to start having migraines with aura and then to change to having them without. Sometimes migraine attacks become much less frequent almost to the point of going away. Sometimes, indeed, they disappear completely. Peter is fortunate in that his attacks became much less frequent after his teens, to the extent that he gets them only once or twice a year now – maybe less. An experience that was very unnerving in childhood is now coloured with some humour.

Peter

I first had them when I was about fourteen years old. They were very bad. I used to get them at least once a week. I'd get strange visions in front of the eyes, and flashing lights. I used to hear strange sounds and have the most peculiar smell under my nose. I couldn't stand any smell, and sounds and light used to put me off as well. It was quite a disruption to my school life. It was difficult to put your mind to your 'O' levels and stuff. I used to get them in the classroom. I didn't know what was going on. The teachers didn't either. I didn't know what had hit me, quite frankly. I used to feel terrible half the time and I didn't know why.

I went to the General Hospital in Birmingham and had tests there. Eventually, three years after I had my first attack I was told I had a form of classical migraine.

One day I was messing about with a pal in the woodwork room when I went into one of these migraines. I was standing in the cloakroom with my head on the table feeling like death warmed up and I looked across and there was another guy standing there looking just as bad as I felt. I said: 'What's the matter with you?'

He said: 'My dad's just died.'

I thought: 'My God – and I'm complaining about these migraines!'

3

Menstrual Migraines

New definitions

Many women link their migraines to their menstrual cycle. However there is a difference between migraines that are period-linked and true menstrual migraines, and the City of London Migraine Clinic has come up with a definition which classifies these two groups of migraines.

True menstrual migraines

These occur regularly between two days prior to bleeding and three days following the outset of bleeding. Only 10 per cent of female migraine patients suffer true menstrual migraines, which occur as a direct result of hormonal changes during menstruation. It is thought by some doctors, but not all, that this group of sufferers can benefit from hormone therapy like the oestrogen patch or other forms of hormone replacement therapy.

Menstrually related migraines

A far larger proportion of women, 35 per cent, suffer from menstrually related migraines. These women regularly get attacks between two days prior to bleeding and three days following the start of bleeding as well as at other times.

Women who suffer from menstrually related migraines usually have other premenstrual symptoms too. These can include fluid retention, bloatedness with associated weight gain, swollen ankles, breast tenderness and a lower resistance to infections and allergies. Fluid retention can be treated with special tablets known as diuretics and these can help migraine. What this group is particularly prey to in relation to migraines is changes in blood sugar. Although women with menstrually related migraines are not likely to benefit from hormone therapy, there are many non-drug ways in which they can help themselves.

Women suffering with migraine without aura are far more likely to be hormonally affected than are women suffering migraine with aura. Some women who suffer from migraine with aura can have attacks without aura which are linked to menstruation.

Treat yourself

So how do you help yourself if you are hormonally affected?

Blood sugar, diet and eating patterns

The number one consideration is blood sugar levels. A drop in blood sugar can cause a migraine at any time of the month, but during menstrually sensitive times migraine sufferers are particularly vulnerable.

Dr Katharina Dalton is renowned for her work on premenstrual syndrome. In her book *Once a Month*, published by Fontana, she explains the fall in blood sugar levels:

> To ensure that the blood sugar always remains within the optimum level we are provided with two regulating mechanisms, an upper and a lower. These prevent the blood sugar level becoming too high (hyperglycaemic) or too low (hypoglycaemic) where we would be in danger of loss of consciousness or death. The blood sugar is maintained by eating carbohydrates, the energy-giving foods, which cover the starches (flour, potatoes, oats, rye and rice) and the sugars. The effect of eating sugars is to cause a rapid rise and rapid drop in the blood sugar level, whereas ingestion of starches brings a more sustained rise. If we eat a large quantity of carbohydrate in one meal the upper regulating mechanism is brought into play, there is a surge of insulin and a valve opens, releasing the extra sugar into the urine. On the other hand if there is a long interval without food and the blood sugar level drops, it may reach the lower regulating mechanism. This causes a sudden outpouring of adrenalin which mobilizes some of the sugar stored in the cells and passes it into the blood so that the blood sugar level is again at the optimum level. However, when sugar is taken from the cells they fill up with water and this is responsible for water retention, bloatedness and weight gain.

> Adrenalin is the hormone which mobilizes the body's defences against 'fright, fight and flight', and this sudden outpouring of adrenalin may be enough to trigger off a sudden fit of irritability, migraine, panic or epilepsy. In others it may cause them to feel weak, shivery, faint or bring on palpitations. On the other hand there are also those fortunate individuals who can manage long fasts, as they are unaware when their blood sugar baseline has been reached, and they get renewed energy from their own sugar stores.

> At this time of the month you must be sure to keep your blood

sugar at the right level and you also need to be mindful of any food that may trigger a migraine. Before a period you should not go more than three hours without food during your waking time. And make sure it is food of the right kind. Proteins are good, as are carbohydrates. Take snacks with you if you are going on a journey and don't know what kind of food will be available. Small, frequent meals are better than large, irregular ones.

Watch out for the busy times. Are you organizing a wedding, or even a dinner party? Is every relative you ever knew spending Christmas with you this year? It is very easy for women to cook large amounts of mouth-watering food for others but to be too busy to eat anything themselves for very long periods. 'I'm rushed off my feet. I haven't got time to stop for a bite,' is the cry of many an anxious hostess. The result is also not uncommon: the guests are downstairs tucking in, happily (if not slightly guiltily) to the culinary extravaganza, while the hostess is upstairs, gripped in the arms of a massive migraine. Don't let it happen to you – at least not now you know!

If you are dieting you might find a Weight Watchers type of diet – including plenty of fresh fruit, vegetables and salad as well as bread, crackers, rice and pasta – will work for you, as it tends to keep the blood sugar levels steady. Always eat breakfast, and if you find that migraines follow a lie-in, it may be because you have gone without food for longer than normal. Try getting up at your normal time to eat something and then going back to bed, or else organize a bedside snack. A good book to help you control your migraines through diet is *The Migraine Guide and Cookbook* by Josie Wentworth, a migraine sufferer herself.

When considering blood sugar, you have to look also at the question of energy, as Dr Dalton points out:

> One must consider not only the interval between meals but the amount of energy exerted during the interval, as the more energy is exerted, the quicker the blood sugar level falls. Overnight fasting is often the cause of a migraine attack on waking, and there are those migraine sufferers who say they cannot sleep long on holidays or at the weekend because they only wake up with a headache. Migraine is likely to occur when the evening meal is followed by some energetic sport or a brisk walk and no further food is taken before retiring to bed.

So physical exertion has a part to play. Obviously you can't eat a big meal and rush off for a game of squash or tennis straight afterwards. But if you know you are going to be playing some sport you can prepare for it. Eat something nutritious an hour or so before, and make absolutely sure you have at least a nutritious snack soon afterwards. The scenario to avoid is the one that has you on the squash court straight after work and then in your kitchen a couple of hours later wondering what to prepare for dinner – with no food having passed your lips since lunchtime.

Just as much as you have to prepare for sports, you have to do the same for sex. Post-coital migraines are not unknown, and they are nothing to do with romance, emotional ardour or giving up cigarettes. It's down to blood sugar. If you are likely to be involved in love-making for some time, take food as well as condoms. Look at it as just another precaution, but make it exotic such as smoked salmon or prawns and fantasize!

It is not just blood sugar that you have to watch out for if you suffer from menstrually related migraines. Foods that you may be able to eat at other times of the month may trigger a migraine during the menstrually sensitive time. The changing levels of the hormones during this period are thought to have this effect. For more information on possible food sensitivities see Chapter 9.

Other treatments

Pyridoxine, or vitamin B6, is very often prescribed for treating premenstrual syndrome; it can be useful in helping with menstrually related migraines. However, you must be careful to keep within the recommended dose as overdosing can cause neurological problems.

Evening primrose oil has also been successfully used by women to counteract the symptoms of premenstrual syndrome. This oil is rich in essential fatty acids and contains in particular gamma linolenic acid (GLA); this substance helps build healthy membranes in every cell of the body and produces prostaglandins which regulate blood pressure, brain function and skin condition. Women suffering from premenstrual syndrome may be low in essential fatty acids and prostaglandin E1; this can lead to an excess of the female hormone prolactin which produces changes in both mood and fluid metabolism. Taking the oil can damp down these symptoms. Many women find that taking both pyridoxine tablets and evening primrose oil capsules daily helps counteract premenstrual symptoms and cuts down the severity of menstrually related migraine attacks.

But how do menstrual migraines affect people's lives? True menstrual migraines have an advantage in that they appear within a limited time span. If your periods are regular, you can predict, within a day or two, when you are going to be struck down. The advantage is that you can often plan to lie low at that time, but better than that, you have the reassurance of knowing the many days in which you will be migraine-free.

With menstrually related migraines this is not so. There are many days in the month which are migraine-possible days. The frequency of attacks, together with not knowing when one is waiting in the wings, can play havoc with people's lives.

Sarah is a professional musician who teaches and plays in concerts. Of course, on the day that her trio were invited to play on the radio she had a massive migraine.

Sarah

I was doing 'O' levels at school, I was under a lot of pressure and feeling very tense. One morning I woke up and I had a blinding pain on the right-hand side of my head. That's the side they normally come on. It was making me sick and I had to take painkillers which at that stage worked. I think that was my first migraine. Since then I've had so many that painkillers really have lost their effect. So I have to wait for them to burn themselves out, which is a very long and arduous process especially if I'm at work.

They are related to periods. Before I get a period I get a lot of headaches. I get them at ovulation time, leading up to the period and during the period itself, and especially at the end of a period. So really there are three weeks out of four which are quite bad and one week when I can be confident that I will actually be clear.

I find that if I do catch the attack in time I can minimize it. But the problem is that most of my migraines start in the middle of the night when I'm asleep. I'm really fast asleep and I'm not aware of the warning signs. They probably start at about four in the morning and I wake up at about seven. There is pain behind both eyes which makes my eyes hurt when I move them around. It makes me feel very sick. Then about three hours later the pain is actually gone from both eyes and concentrated on one side of the head. By this time I'm usually sick, which creates a problem taking painkillers, because within a very few minutes of taking something I'm sick again and so they come back.

My doctor has prescribed Stemetil, which I take, but to be honest it really doesn't help at all. Even swallowing a little pill like that makes me sick again.

The pain settles on the right-hand side of my head and it keeps on all day. It seems to get particularly unpleasant at teatime. It reaches a crescendo of pain when I can't bear looking at any lights or the television or hearing any noises at all. I've got to be in a darkened room.

I would be out of action a lot if I allowed myself. There's many a time when I've got to do a concert in terrible pain – really I just battle on if

I can. Music is very difficult – the sound can jar on the pain very much. I'm a flautist, which involves a lot of blowing, and that seems to aggravate it.

Last year my flute trio was invited to play on Radio One and this was a tremendous opportunity. But typically I woke up that morning with a terrible migraine. I just had to stuff myself full of painkillers without exceeding the stated dose, and I don't know how I got through it. Luckily there's caffeine in the Solpadeine tablets I take, and that seems to keep me going. I had to play with sunglasses on because my eyes were so bad. I play a lot by memory – the physical action of trying to read a lot of dots when you've got a migraine is impossible. I over-compensate when I'm ill and I drive myself even harder because I know that I'm not functioning as well. The performance went very well.

Saturday is the favourite day for my migraines to come – that's a very busy day for me because I give music lessons all day and there is usually a concert in the evening, so I ready can't relax at all. I've got to keep popping out in the middle of lessons to be sick. Sometimes I have to pop out in the interval during a concert to be sick.

I also sing in a choir. I've got a very loud voice and I'm somebody who always goes at everything 100 per cent. I always give my maximum effort. I think that might be one of the problems. When I sing in this choir on a Friday night I sing really loudly and have a jolly good time. But then, as I say, Saturday is the most likely day for waking up with one of these migraines.

Holidays can be an awful problem for migraine patients. The journey itself can set off a migraine, and there's nothing worse than having a severe attack when you're a long way from familiar and convenient surroundings. Joanna describes such an attack; her eating pattern may also strike a chord with many migraine sufferers.

Joanna
We went to an island off Ibiza and it was in the middle of the summer. It was very hot. We were supposed to be going to what was termed in the brochure a 'lovely villa'. It was more like a chicken hut. We had a very long journey there – first the plane, after which we had to wait for about two hours in the heat and then travel over on the ferry to this place. The migraine just started coming on and I had to go and lie down in the bedroom. There were slits for windows and bars up at them and my husband had to race off to get a doctor because I was having convulsions. I was hallucinating. My husband said I kept saying strange things. I was talking mumbo-jumbo really. That was probably a combination of the heat as well as the migraine. My son kept running down to get ice packs

out of the fridge to cool me down. Eventually the doctor came and gave me an injection. That attack lasted about two days. Eventually they moved us to a better villa and I settled down. But that was pretty horrendous.

My migraines began when I started my periods at the age of fourteen. I get them at ovulation time or period time – sometimes both. A typical attack starts when I can feel the head coming on. It's always on one side – usually over my eye. It gets worse and worse until I just feel terribly sick and dizzy. I try and ride over them, but if it's a full-blown migraine I can't. I have to go to bed. I vomit terribly and I have very bad diarrhoea. It seems to go through my whole system. It's as though it starts in the head and works its way right down the whole body. It usually lasts two full days – forty-eight hours. The pain is so bad I'm head banging – I hit my head against the wall. I don't take anything for the sickness because in a funny sort of way it seems to be a relief to be sick. I'm just retching and retching, but the pain in the head is so bad that the sickness doesn't worry me too much. Once the pain has gone it takes me about a day to come round, because I feel very weak and my legs are like jelly. Usually the following day I'm fine – back to normal.

I have noticed that just before I have one I feel extremely well, energetic and euphoric. That can also happen when I've just had one. My husband calls it being on a high.

I've studied all the food allergies. I don't eat chocolate and full fat cheese and that sort of thing. I am a sensible eater. I eat lots and lots of salads, I watch my weight anyway – I'm quite slim and I want to stay that way. So I don't eat a lot of stodge. During the day I just snack. I have cereal or toast at breakfast. Then I don't have anything substantial at lunch, and I never sit down to it. I work part-time, and when I finish I go and exercise my dog immediately. I'd probably take an apple with me up on the moor and make that do, and maybe have a little cottage cheese when I come home. But then I do eat quite a lot in the evening.

Alison thinks she has a migraine personality. She says she is the type of person who is very conscientious and has to do everything as well as she possibly can. As a child she used to be travel sick. She started having migraines in her teens and had them right throughout pregnancy. She gets them at ovulation time and any time leading up to her period plus the week of her period. She has tried osteopathy and acupuncture, but without success. Feverfew made it worse, but she finds preparations with caffeine helpful and says she always eats little and often. The migraines have seriously curtailed her life.

Alison

It makes it very difficult to plan or arrange things. I used to keep goats. Not very many – just enough to keep my family and one or two neighbours in milk. But I had to give that up because I was being ill so often and it was too much to expect other people to keep taking over.

At the moment I am taking Cafergot when I have the migraine. I also take Sanomigran and amitriptyline every night. At the moment I am taking quite a lot. I've had a bad patch. I think I am hitting the change of life, so my hormones are all mixed up.

I get severe migraines once a month, typically on the first day of my period but sometimes the day before. I usually awake with one. If I take medication in time I can either avert it or it will only last until about four o'clock. If I don't get it in time, it's a twenty-four-hour job.

It will start with a pain over the left eye. It's a sharp pain and quite often it pulsates along with my heartbeat. Sometimes I get palpitations as well. It's a rhythmic sort of pain which goes along the side of my head, down my ear, and sometimes down my neck and right down into my shoulders. I feel generally ill, aching all over and a little bit nauseated. This usually builds up until I am sick, although I do take Stemetil. I'm usually sick five or six times. I can't sleep or anything. I just have to lie there with my head under a pillow. Then it will gradually start dying down towards the late evening. I'll be able to sleep that night, and by morning it's usually gone.

I can't stand light. I dislike sound, but it's not as bad as light. I find people walking across the floor and shaking the bed uncomfortable. I can't eat or drink anything because I start being sick. I try and keep drinking until I'm sick, because I'm sick so much that there's nothing to bring up – it's easier if you've got something in there. Retching makes the pain worse. Any movement aggravates the pain, so I try and keep as still as I can. I also try and do yoga relaxation and meditation.

My family keep popping in to see if I want anything. If all they get is a grunt they know I'm all right. I'm conscious of them being there but when the pain is really bad it hurts to talk. They're very understanding. At first my husband felt so frustrated and helpless because he couldn't do anything that he used to get cross with me. That of course didn't help. But now he's very understanding. He's got so used to me having it and he's been with me to various doctors. I've tried just about everything there is.

Although I'm out of action one or two days in a month, half the month I'm not working at full strength. I haven't got a migraine, but I haven't not got one either. I find it hard to concentrate or plan anything. It takes me all my strength to go from day to day doing the basics. If I *have to do something out of the ordinary it throws me and I get panicky about it.*

I am very lucky with my present doctors. If I have a really bad migraine – I've had a few which won't respond to the Cafergot and have gone on for two or three days – they are prepared to come out and give me morphine. To know you've got that to fall back on if you're desperate is marvellous. I'm very lucky to find a doctor like that, I think.

Denise's migraines are very much of the menstrually related kind in that they can come at ovulation time, just before, during or after her periods. She often gets them twice a month. She feels that over the years the vomiting has caused her other problems.

Denise
The headache lasts for twenty-four hours and the vomiting sometimes goes on for about twelve hours. I usually end up on my knees in the bathroom with my head over the toilet. Also my bowels go very loose. It's as though my system is just throwing everything out at both ends.

I've been in hospital and had a scan. They say I've had an ulcer which has healed. I think it was all the vomiting over the years which caused it. I still get pain in my stomach. It's like I've got no lining left in it. I've never been a stomach sufferer. It's all down to the vomiting.

As you can imagine, I dread every month coming around. It's pointless taking a tablet as I can't keep it down. I've tried taking tablets when I've felt the aura, but all I ever succeed in doing is delaying it – and then it will creep up on me or I'll wake up with it. The thing I hate most is not the actual migraine but knowing I'm going to get it. When the aura comes over I know there's no turning back. I just can't describe the dread I feel.

I must just add that after the headache is over and I've recovered from the weakness, I can go right through the house as though I'm regenerated. I sometimes wonder whether it's just the sheer relief that the headache has gone.

I remember the Garden Festival at Liverpool. A neighbour and I had bought tickets. I took my little girl. On the way I felt this migraine coming on. I was sick when I got off the bus. Then we had to get on another bus. I spent the whole day lying on the grass. I was lying there and everybody was milling around me. It was a big festival – a big tourist attraction – and I was lying flat out on the grass from early in the morning until six o'clock that night. I was sick once or twice. I remember staggering about. It was the one thing I dreaded – being stranded somewhere with a migraine.

I know it's an awful thing to say but sometimes I think it would be better to be disabled completely in a wheelchair, because then you know your limitations. But with migraine, in between you're just expected to get on with your life as normal. I think the least sympathetic people are doctors: it doesn't kill you, so you just have to live with it.

4
What's in a Womb?

Pregnancy

Roughly eighty per cent of women migraine sufferers do not get an attack during pregnancy. These are usually patients who suffer migraine without aura, and the migraines tend to disappear around the fourth month. However, many women suffer worse migraines in the first three months of pregnancy before they improve. This is most likely to happen in women whose migraines are menstrually related. The reason could be that the rise and fall of the hormones during the menstrual cycle is replaced during pregnancy by a rise in the level of oestrogenic hormones. Or, as Dr Marcia Wilkinson writes in *Migraine and Headaches*, it may be due to biochemical changes that occur during pregnancy. Blood sugar may play a part, too – in pregnant women the blood sugar level is higher than normal, and this may help to prevent attacks.

Unfortunately there is a price to pay. Many women who experience this relief during pregnancy wind up with an all-singing, all-dancing migraine attack after the baby is born.

However, nothing is true for everybody: some women get their first migraine during pregnancy, while others continue to suffer attacks all the way through. These women have a real problem because so many of the drugs used to prevent or treat an attack must be avoided during pregnancy. Drugs taken by the mother can cross the placenta and enter the baby's bloodstream. *The British Medical Association Guide to Medicine and Drugs* states the position clearly. The first three months of pregnancy are the most critical. During this time drugs can affect the development of the baby's organs, which could lead to congenital malformation. Very severe defects can result in miscarriage. From the fourth to the sixth month of pregnancy some drugs may retard the growth of the foetus and also result in a low birth weight. During the final three months risks include breathing difficulties in the new born baby. Also some drugs can affect labour, causing it to be premature, delayed or prolonged.

In addition, the *BMA Guide* warns, caution has to be taken with drugs while breast-feeding. The milk-producing glands in the breast are surrounded by a network of fine blood vessels. Small molecules of substances such as drugs pass from the blood into the milk. This means that a breast-fed baby may receive small doses of whatever drugs the mother is taking. In many cases this is not a problem because the amount of drug that passes into the milk is too small to have any significant effect on the baby. However, some drugs can produce unwanted side-effects in the baby.

So the minute you have the slightest inkling that you may be pregnant – or, better than that, if you are planning to start a family – go and see your doctor about the medication you take either on a daily basis or to treat an attack.

Two drugs that should not be taken during pregnancy are ergotamine and methysergide. Also, if you are pregnant you should not take aspirin or propranolol without consulting your doctor. But this list is not exhaustive so it is important to ask your doctor about any medication you are taking.

The story of Angela is horrendous. Very much more is known about drugs and pregnancy these days. Angela's traumatic experience probably altered the course of her life.

Angela

One Sunday morning I awoke feeling absolutely terrible. I felt as if I was being pinned to the bed by my head and a dreadful weight was holding it there. I didn't know what was wrong. When I went to get out of bed I was violently sick. My mum had heard me get up. She came out, took one look at me and said: 'You've got a migraine.'

I was seventeen years old at the time, and as far back as I could remember my mother had had migraines. I felt as if I was having bricks piled on top of my head one after another and they were slowly being driven in. The pressure was everywhere. There seemed to be no escape and I couldn't speak – every time I tried I would get sick.

I started to get migraines once a week and then they increased to twice weekly. Each migraine would last twenty-four hours and it would take me a day to get over it. So you can see that I was having no life at all. I started taking Cafergot daily to keep myself on an even keel. Without it I just could not cope with the pain and the sickness. The doctor knew the amount of Cafergot I was taking, prescribed it freely and did not seem unduly concerned.

When I became pregnant I was over the moon. I asked at the hospital if I should continue with the Cafergot, and they said I could providing I kept the dose down. One Saturday morning when I was six months pregnant I felt strange pains around my tummy and back. They were not severe, so I didn't worry. But by the evening the pain had got so bad that my husband rushed out to a phone box to call the doctor. While he was gone there was this loud pop like a champagne cork coming out of a bottle and my waters broke – everywhere! I was terrified. The baby's kicks started coming very quickly and very hard, and then, all of a sudden, they stopped. I knew my baby was dead. When I got to the hospital I was attached to a drip and told that as the baby was dead I would have to do all the work myself. I was given no painkillers in any shape or form. The joyless labour took twelve hours but seemed endless, and I can tell you it is the only pain I have ever had comparable to the severity of migraine. I was twenty-three at the time.

I was determined not to let my migraines interfere with my life. We had been told we could try for a family again but to wait a few months first. So I got on with living – working, entertaining and going out. Possibly this was the time in my life I was taking the most Cafergot – but again, with my doctor's knowledge and approval.

When I was twenty-five I became pregnant again. I was advised not to work this time but I could keep on with the Cafergot, so long as I kept the dosage low. This I did and all progressed well for the first four and a half months. Then I woke up one morning to the tell-tale signs of a miscarriage. Once again I wound up in hospital, on a drip, slowly, painfully and single-handedly giving birth to a dead baby.

We then moved house, which brought me into the district of my old family doctor who had looked after my mum through her migraines. I had been getting some pain in my calf muscles. I wanted to get pregnant again, but this doctor said he wasn't happy about my taking the ergotamine. He sent me to see a neurologist. After examination, the neurologist said he couldn't feel any of the pulse points in my legs. He thought I had a huge build up of ergotamine in my system, which was causing the legs to go into spasm and not allowing the blood to flow properly. The condition was reversible, but only if I came off ergotamine. I was quickly admitted to hospital

Within twenty-four hours of coming off I was in the most excruciating pain and being sick all the time. I was also being put through different tests to make sure that it was migraine I was suffering from. One test was lumbar puncture, which entails putting a needle into your spine and drawing fluid off for testing. You get a very bad headache afterwards. This was added to the migraine, the sickness and the headache caused by ergotamine withdrawal. I wish I could describe it but there aren't the words. All I can tell you is that the agony lasted two weeks.

I eventually recovered and returned home off the ergotamine. But now I had another problem. I could not conceive. I started to get desperate. All my friends seemed to be having babies. Every time I entered a room where my pregnant friends were chatting, the conversation stopped for fear of hurting me. I began to feel very isolated. My husband and I went overboard during the next four years with hormone injections, fertility charts and fertility drugs – all to no avail.

I was admitted to hospital to see why I wasn't conceiving. They found that since my last miscarriage one of my fallopian tubes had broken off and I only had a 50/50 chance each month of becoming pregnant. In the meantime the fertility drugs had made my migraines worse. So here I was – handicapped in my ability to have a baby and unable to live a normal life in every other way. Without the ergotamine my migraines were out of control. I decided that I would forget about having a baby and go back on the ergotamine to control my migraines.

Within no time at all I became pregnant! I was told at the outset that I could miscarry. This third pregnancy was a nightmare. I was off the ergotamine and being sick all the time. There was no joy in the fact that I was at last pregnant because I didn't think for one minute I would keep the baby since I was so ill all the time. I had a lot of medical help with this pregnancy, but I believe it came too late for me. Six months into the pregnancy the baby died in my womb. The hospital registrar cried as she broke the news to me, and she sat with me through the twenty-two hours it took to deliver my dead child.

Angela's marriage eventually broke up and although she is now happily remarried she has a very restricted work and social life. She has no children of her own and she is still on ergotamine.

Hysterectomy

Many women are convinced that their migraines are somehow linked to their wombs. If the migraines are menstrually related it seems a logical conclusion. But removing the womb does not seem to provide any answers to migraine attacks. The hormones that control menstruation come from the hypothalamus and the hypothalamus remains even when the womb has been removed. The fact is that just as many women suffer worse attacks after a hysterectomy as are improved by the operation and an equal number experience only a temporary change. So a hysterectomy should only be contemplated for gynaecological reasons.

Having a hysterectomy does not have quite the same effect on a woman's body chemistry as does the menopause. In her book *Once a Month*, Dr Katharina Dalton explains why:

In a natural menopause, the changes are very gradual over several years, with a slow closing down of the menstrual clock and shrinking of the ovaries and womb, but in an artificial menopause the changes are sudden and only affect the womb and/or the ovaries, leaving the menstrual clock intact.

All goes well after the operation for some months but then those who previously suffered from the premenstrual syndrome will find that the usual cyclic symptoms return. Often it is the husband who is the first to notice it and he will try to remind the wife of what is happening. Or she may recognize the tell-tale headache, which previously ushered in a period and now assumes the proportion of a prostrating migraine.

Dr Dalton adds:

While carrying out a nationwide survey into the hormonal factors in migraine in women in 1975, it was noted that it was those women with a history of premenstrual syndrome who stated that the severity of their migraine had been increased by the hysterectomy. Their three-month charts giving the precise timing of migraine attacks confirmed the attacks were still occurring cyclically.

Brenda was so convinced that a hysterectomy would cure her of her incapacitating migraines that against the advice of her GP and her migraine specialist, she went privately to a gynaecologist and paid to have her womb removed. She had no respite from attacks at all. 'The day after the operation I woke up with a migraine and I just howled my eyes out,' she says. The nurse told her: 'We've had people like you before. We had another woman who went everywhere and tried everything. She ended up a drug addict.'

Brenda

I have diagnosed myself as having common migraines. I first started having headaches when I was fifteen and my mother took me to a doctor. He said I should go to a neurological hospital but I never did. Then I went into the ATS [army]. I had headaches but I could get rid of them. I'd have an aspirin and lie down. But I did notice that I had them frequently. I always felt unwell.

I was thirty when I sought help again, and it was diagnosed as migraine. I've been quite severe since then. I've always got a headache. I have more days unwell than I have well. When I was younger I could probably cope better because although I had them frequently I was a very competent person and I helped run a business. I love business – I love working hard and organizing. I ran a busy fast-food restaurant with my husband. I had to go to bed when I had an attack. A glass of water would be beside my bed. I had nausea and I was very sensitive to noise and I'd have a pounding headache. I can't go in these shops where they've got music on. My attacks always lasted twenty-four hours. I would get up the next day feeling very unwell, but I'd get to business because I had to – which is good for you, ready. I'm retired now. When we sold up I thought I wouldn't have these problems and I'd be better – but quite frankly I think I've been worse. I've got to the point where I am either building up to one or I've got one or I'm getting over one and then I'm back into another one.

My mother had migraine. She called it bilious attacks. I can only remember her with a great big bottle of Aspro, in bed, vomiting violently and saying she was going to die. I was only a child and I used to think: 'Please God, don't let her die.' When I was young I did think she was going to die. But my mum out-grew it at the change. This is why I got it into my head that it would go with my periods. I have a sister who has it as well. I can remember my aunt on my father's side wandering around with an ice pack on her head. She had constant headaches, so obviously she also had migraines. I used to think she was nutty. Now I think maybe God is punishing me.

When I was forty-four or forty-five I thought if I could get rid of my periods I would be all right. I had a hysterectomy when I didn't need it. I paid for it privately and woke up the day after the operation with a migraine.

The funniest thing is, when I am well – and it isn't that very often – I am so well it's unbelievable. I open the windows and I want to sing. The hoover is buzzing away early in the morning. Life is so different. I can dance. I'm as alive as anything. I don't feel sixty-five. I feel like a young girl. I can be the life and soul of the party. I think: 'Gosh, other people must be like this always.' They don't know how lucky they are. If I have two days like that I think maybe I'm over it now. Maybe it's the end of the migraines. But it's not. The next day I'm in bed flaked out. People don't know that side of you. I'm very conscious of it and I don't like people to know that I'm not well. When people ask, I say: 'Fine. I'm fine' when I feel like death. I don't want people to know, because I don't want people to think: 'Oh, she's one of those.'

Every now and again I get really depressed and weepy. I'm really down but I know I have everything to be happy for – except for the migraines and they dominate my life. Nobody wants to be unwell. Nobody has any sympathy when you're unwell. You don't want sympathy. You want understanding.

Currently Brenda is handling her migraines by taking Migril (an ergotamine-based drug) at the first sign of an attack. This often aborts the attack.

I sometimes take as many as three a week, which I know is not good. But, you know, I play bridge with a friend who also suffers from migraines and he takes Migril every day. When I told him I thought he was mad he said he was seventy-four years old and he'd rather have what was left and go early. That's true, isn't it? With what's left you want quality, don't you?

Amy was advised to have a hysterectomy for her migraines when she was in South Africa. Her attacks have subsequently got worse.

Amy

I have been having migraines for a long time but they have only been diagnosed recently. When I first started having them I was told they were tension headaches or I was depressed – all that rubbish. I have common migraine. But I have also been told that I have trigeminal neuralgia which sometimes goes together with it.

My migraines terrify me. I have terrible nausea. I yawn a tremendous amount. I have body weakness and I get hot and cold. I smell things that aren't there and I am extremely sensitive to light and sound. I find it difficult to talk. I cease to function. I have daymares. You know what I mean? I see frightening things. I see pictures jump around on the wall. I once saw an old man sitting on the other side of the room.

They have ripped out my insides because of my migraines. I had a hysterectomy done when I was thirty-nine. I am forty-six now. They seemed to think that the hysterectomy would do the trick. It had a terrible effect on me. It made me feel very ill, and it traumatized me beyond belief because the one thing I'd always wanted was children. Psychologically it made me feel like death. The migraines have got worse. I get very little remission at all now. I am in constant pain.

It's made my life a total misery. I haven't worked for about two years. My close friends are good but a lot of people find continuous illness very difficult. That's why a lot of people turn away. They think you're deranged. They think it's a psychological thing which is even more isolating. A lot of doctors think that, too.

5

The Other Big 'M'

Menopause

There was a time when, if you were a young unmarried woman and you went to your doctor complaining of headaches or other nebulous pains he would assure you that all your problems would end once you were married. Whether the doctor (this advice almost always came from the male of the species) had some sort of touching faith in the healing powers of the love of a good man, or whether he knew very well that a woman, once married and with children, has no time to be ill depended, I dare say, on the perception of the particular doctor.

These days very few doctors would say that – instead, women migraine sufferers are assured that all will be well come the menopause. No one wants to grow old, but it is surprising how many female migraineurs look forward to the change.

The fact is that many women do cease to have migraines once they have completed their menopause. But some suffer more frequent or severe attacks during the menopausal years and after, while others have the illness diagnosed for the first time during the menopause. A small paragraph in the Winter 1989/90 *Newsletter of the British Migraine Association* carried the following information:

> A group from Brazil studied the relationship between migraine and the menopause. They found that in their small sample of twenty-three patients with migraine only seven had less frequent attacks after menopause. In nine of the women, the frequency remained unchanged or increased. Migraine was diagnosed for the first time in four menopausal women. They found that other forms of headache were also more frequent in the women they studied, probably reflecting the higher prevalence of headache in the general population of this age and sex.

If your migraines are menstrually related there is a good chance that they will improve or cease after the menopause. This is because they may be caused by the hormonal changes that take place in the body during the menstrual cycle. A clear explanation of the female sex hormones appears in *The British Medical Association's Guide to*

Medicine and Drugs.

There are two types of female sex hormones, oestrogens and progesterone. In women these are secreted by the ovaries from puberty until after the menopause. Additional oestrogens and progesterone are produced by the placenta during pregnancy. Small amounts of oestrogens are also produced in the adrenal glands.

Oestrogens are responsible for the development of female sexual characteristics including breast development, growth of pubic hair and widening of the pelvis. Progesterone acts on the lining of the uterus and prepares it for the implantation of the fertilized egg. It is also important for the maintenance of pregnancy. On a monthly basis, levels of oestrogens and progesterone fluctuate, producing the menstrual cycle.

A fall in the level of oestrogens and progesterone occurs naturally after the menopause, when the menstrual cycle ceases. The sudden reduction in levels of oestrogen often causes distressing symptoms including sweating, hot flushes, dryness of the vagina and mood changes.

This reduction in the levels of oestrogen and progesterone can bring an end to the attacks of some, but by no means all, migraine sufferers. If your mother or your aunt suffered migraines and then said goodbye to them at the menopause, there is every chance that your migraines will end there too. However, bear in mind that the menopause takes place over a period of time – usually between five to seven years. It can happen as early as thirty-five or as late as fifty-six, but on average it will begin between the ages of forty-eight and fifty-two. The form it takes also varies from woman to woman. Usually the periods grow further apart, and when they do come they are scantier and last a shorter time. But for some women the cycles are shorter and the periods may be much heavier than before. For other women menstruation just ceases.

In the same way that as young girls we went through the biological and emotional upheaval of puberty, we have to go through the menopause – often with less sympathy and understanding. At puberty you are growing up. At the menopause you are growing old. For many women it is a time of adjustment. You say goodbye to your periods, but maybe also to your children and to a part of your life that was very important to you. You look in the mirror, and wrinkles that must belong to somebody else stare back at you. You look out of the window and see your daughter in an outfit that you would like to be able to wear – or at least to have worn if only it had been around in your time. There are a lot of goodbyes. So why shouldn't one be migraine?

For some women the menopausal years can be the most trying, certainly as far as their migraines are concerned. A woman who knew that her migraines would come around the time of her periods had some form of security – at least she knew when she would be free. During the menopause this can change – with devastating results. Deborah's is a very sad and moving story. She had just 'come out' of an attack when I interviewed her and she wept as she told some of her story.

Deborah

You probably wouldn't believe me. They're so bad that quite honestly I just want to die. I know that sounds melodramatic but I'm not a melodramatic person. It started after my daughter was born eighteen years ago. The worst thing is when you know you're getting one. It's like a time bomb. You know that within seconds or minutes or even a couple of hours you are going to explode. It's like a monster in your body coming out. It's the most awful pain imaginable – worse than giving birth and that's bad enough. Also I get sick and have diarrhoea, and every time I am sick or have diarrhoea the pain increases in intensity.

When the pain first starts I lie down. Then I feel sick and throw up. Then it goes to a further stage which is when I start pacing about. I can't bear light. My neck hurts and my head feels too big for my body. I have to have someone pacing the floor with me. I can't cope on my own any more. Somebody has to come with me with a bucket because of the sickness and diarrhoea and I can't see what I'm doing. I have to have my eyes completely covered. It's as if I'm blind. My husband calls it doing a macabre dance together. He follows me around with a bucket. He has to take his shoes off because I can't stand any sound. I end up actually on the floor at the third stage. I'm curled up wishing I was dead. The pain in my eye is dreadful and the photophobia is extreme. I feel like an animal because if you don't get to the toilet in time – you know. But I don't think animals have it as bad. Afterwards I feel if it wasn't for my family . . .

They were always once a month when I had my periods. I'm forty-seven and my periods are rare now. For the last eighteen months I've never known when I'm having an attack. Before, although it was agony, I could put that part of my life into a box. I can't do that any more. Over the years the doctors have used me as a guinea pig, for everything. Fringe medicines, ordinary medicine – I've tried all the drugs – I could write a book on it. Now all I take is a Cafergot suppository when the attack starts. Nothing else works. It doesn't ease the pain but it accelerates everything. It's like a speeded up film. Instead of lasting days the attack lasts hours.

I am a Christian and I try and find solace in it, but I can't say I do. I have had some wonderful support from a priest who once came and witnessed me in an attack – which is more than a doctor has ever done. The reason I am telling you this is because there have been a couple of times when I have gone into a terrible black hole of despair and I haven't felt like living again after it. I had to go and tell somebody who wasn't the family because I didn't want my husband to know. He does now. It frightened me because I can remember after one terrible attack thinking: 'I am in this black hole and I don't want to come out.' I felt that it was pointless going on and I might as well finish it all now.

It took hold of me. It happened twice. They were coupled with what I had been through during the migraines. It was too traumatic for me to handle. I wanted to take my own life and that terrified me. If I had had anything to take it with I probably would have done. Normally, after an attack, although I still feel terribly ill I start having a little bit of hope. I start glancing towards the next thing I want to do when I feel well enough. I start thinking of ways to climb out of it. I'm a terrific climber-outer. But on these two occasions I didn't want to. I was deadly cold and I seemed to feel a blackness all around me. I didn't want to experience another migraine and I knew I would and I just felt swamped. I wanted to sink peacefully into oblivion. It was since the menopause when I could no longer shut away the migraines in a box.

I went to this priest and I said: 'You've got to help me.' He came and just talked and helped me enormously. He didn't say the things that I desperately didn't want him to say like: 'It's in God's hands.' And, you know, 'It's for a purpose.' I didn't want anything like that. And he didn't. He didn't say holier than thou things. He was just so ordinary. He made me a cup of tea and just listened.

The other thing is the awful feeling of guilt. Migraines have practically ruined my life. When the kids were little my husband had to come home from work. I've got virtually no social life. It would have broken up another marriage, I think. I've been brought home from numerous meetings and social events. I don't go to social events any more. I feel I'm ruining other people's lives as well as my own. I've been lucky to keep a job. I'm a nursery nurse. This one's a fairly new job. I don't tell them I have migraines. I make up anything. I say I have an earache or a virus. I don't want people to know. I don't know why. The funny thing is that it's so hidden. People keep telling me how well I look and I hate it. I think: 'If only you could have seen me.' I've got this awful thing inside my head. Sometimes I want people to know what it is like.

I've got a lovely, lovely husband and wonderful children. Also I've taken up an Open University degree in psychology. I feel I have to do a lot in between attacks. Migraine people are fighters.

Annabel, who has suffered from migraines since childhood, held down a demanding job in the National Health Service where she was a lecturer on personnel and administration. This was no mean task since some of her worst symptoms were nausea, sickness, temporary loss of memory and speech difficulties. She would often experience them during the course of a lecture, so she resorted to tricks. One was to make herself vomit in between lectures, as she knew this would forestall any such occurrence later while she was talking. But she would return from the loo feeling weak and shaky and worried about losing the thread of her lecture. She relied heavily on notes. However, since the menopause her migraine attacks became progressively more frequent and in 1985 she decided that she had run out of tricks. When she was just over forty she took early retirement because of ill health.

Annabel

I seem to get all sorts of attacks. I can feel euphoric or I can feel ill just before it starts. I only very occasionally get a massive headache now, but I always get a feeling of tightness in my head. I get this awful ill feeling in my body. When I wake up in the morning my legs ache – it's almost impossible to get moving. Sometimes I pass a lot of urine. Sometimes I get diarrhoea. This ill feeling can go on for two or three days. Nowadays I can get the symptoms of a new attack before I've finished the old one. They leave me feeling absolutely drained. I've got to the stage now when I have about a couple of days a week when I'm feeling reasonable.

I've been through just about everything in the book – pills, tests, the lot. I had an electroencephalograph [where the electrical activity of the brain is amplified and recorded on paper]. I've had a brain scan, urine and blood tests. They've all come up with nothing. Just before Christmas my GP sent me to a neurologist. I'd been to see him before. He examined me and said that with my type of migraine he could do nothing for me. I asked him about sumatriptan. He said: 'What are you talking about?' He would have me believe that he hadn't heard that Glaxo were testing this new drug. He said: 'Tell me about it. I must keep my eyes open for it.' I'm afraid I felt patronized and very, very cross.

Migraines rule my life. I can't work now. I have no children and I don't know how I would have coped if I had. Social engagements are a nightmare because I never know when I am going to have to cancel.

My half sister who was much older than me was mentally handicapped. She lived with us for a while. She used to have days of feeling ill, and of course with being mentally handicapped it was difficult to tell, but my husband can see in me the same symptoms as she displayed. Nobody ever diagnosed it but he thinks she had migraines – certainly abdominal ones.

At the moment I am on anti-depressants, just 75mg of Prothiaden a night. They haven't done anything for the migraine but they make me happier about them – I think!

Hormone replacement therapy

These days menopausal women do have an ally in the shape of hormone replacement therapy. The hormones that start to go missing and cause unwanted menopausal symptoms can be replaced artificially by means of pills, patches and implants. Probably the most important service that HRT provides is in counteracting osteoporosis – brittle bone disease. But it is not all plain sailing for the migraine patient. If your migraines are likely to end when the hormones in your system lessen, then replacing those hormones is likely to counteract that effect. Indeed, HRT can aggravate migraines in some patients, which makes it a difficult option. You may find that you would rather put up with the hot flushes and night sweats than suffer migraine – but what of osteoporosis? It is very difficult to predict at fifty what your bones are going to be like at seventy.

Diet and the amount of calcium intake is very important and so is exercise. You could try looking at the family. Genetics is one guide, but it is not fail-safe as there are other variables – your own health over the years, for instance. Do your mother and her sisters still walk tall, or are their backs bending considerably? It can be an indication of things to come. It is important to book a consultation with your doctor. There are so many different forms of HRT with varying hormonal brews that he or she may eventually be able to find one that gives your bones protection without upsetting the migraine apple cart too much (if at all). However, it is worth knowing that if HRT aggravates the migraines, once you are taken off the treatment the symptoms usually subside. Incidentally, women who suffer migraine for the first time at the menopause can often be helped by HRT.

Helen
It started four years ago when I was thirty-eight, I was working full-time and feeling sick all day. I couldn't eat much and I lost one and a half stone in three months. A week before my period was due I had these strange feelings in my head. It was like something being pulled tight around my head. My vision kept going blurred and out of focus. I had

flashing lights, zigzags and funny blotches in front of my eyes. I would feel a bit dizzy. The room wouldn't actually go round, it sort of moved – swayed. I found it frightening. My head would feel so heavy at times that I could hardly hold it up. My neck and shoulders would be so tight that they hurt. This lasted for a whole week before my period.

I felt such a nit going to the doctor's and describing these funny things. I sat there and I thought he was going to say: 'You're mad.' But he turned around and said: 'You've got migraine.' I thought: 'Thank goodness he's given it a name.' I said that I didn't have headaches but he said: 'You've got all the rest.'

After three months the pattern changed. I'd get the disturbed vision from about the third day of my period to about the twentieth. I worked in a cleaners doing repairs and alterations. Sometimes I couldn't see what I was unpicking and I'd get worried. My vision would go blurred and it would come back and then go again. That's how my vision was all the time. If I saw any stripes it played havoc with me, and I couldn't bear any bright colours. I couldn't go shopping. The town was too much. Every shop I went into had bright colours. The brightness of the packages used to be agony. It was really bad. But all that seems to have settled now.

After the doctor diagnosed migraine he advised me to give up the trigger foods. It got so that every time I had a migraine I'd blame it on such and such a food and wouldn't eat it any more. I went through a phase of hardly eating anything but I still got the migraines.

I had a weekend when the pain was so bad I just sat with the curtains closed. My husband said: 'You're not going to work tomorrow', and that was it. I gave up working. I'd had enough. The doctor suggested complete rest. He had been trying me on all sorts of tablets and none of them had worked.

I went to see a gynaecologist who said: 'Your oestrogen is too high.' He gave me pills to lower the oestrogen. It didn't work. I still had the migraines just as bad.

In April last year I saw an advertisement in the paper announcing an Amarant Trust meeting. [The Amarant Trust is a charity that has been set up to promote a greater knowledge and understanding of the menopause]. It mentioned migraine, so I went along. They showed a video which listed all the menopause symptoms. I had nearly every one of them. I spoke to one of the women there and she suggested I try the patch. My doctor agreed, so I was put on an oestrogen patch with progesterone tablets to take. After about two days I felt great. I had loads of energy. The blurred vision went and so did a lot of the other symptoms. I still got migraines but it took the edge off and I was able to cope with them.

After about four months I started to get hot flushes and the tiredness started coming back again. The doctor put me on a higher dose. I've been on it for about six months and I've been a lot better. I still get migraines, but if I take a migraine tablet it gets rid of them quickly. Also I don't get them so often and they're not as bad.

I work from home now, making curtains for a shop. The other day I left the house and got in the car. When I got down the road I suddenly felt really sick. My stomach churned over and I felt all shaky. I thought: 'Shall I go back?' And then I thought: 'No you won't. You carry on.' By the time I got to town I realized it was the beginning of a migraine. My head started to go tight and I felt really sick. I was shaking. When I got to the shop I asked for some water and took some Migraleve. An hour later I was fine.

HRT did not work quite so well for Barbara. A local league table-tennis player and international referee for the game, Barbara had a hysterectomy at the age of thirty-eight. She had suffered severe migraines since her early twenties.

Barbara
When it first started I lost my sight completely when I was crossing the road. Fortunately I was with somebody because it frightened the living daylights out of me. The visual disturbance then became a blob which grew bigger and I would go tingly.

I'd get nausea but not be sick, and I would get a dreadful pain usually in my left eye. It was as if somebody was standing there with a knife and just stabbing me in the eye – to a lovely rhythm, of course! This lasted for about five or six hours and I would feel dreadful afterwards.

After she had a hysterectomy, Barbara's migraines became a lot better, but she started to suffer badly from hot flushes and so was prescribed an oestrogen preparation called Prempak. These tablets very quickly resulted in the worst migraine Barbara had experienced for years. It lasted for nearly a week and no tablets she took could touch the pain.

I was really banging my head against the bedpost. It was such a shock after having manageable migraines for so many years. The doctor told me not to worry and that there were plenty of other HRT tablets we could try. I was put on Cyclo-Progynova and I was also on propranolol for the migraines. This seemed to do the trick – no hot flushes and no migraines. But what I did do was put on a stone in a month. I was told by a nurse that this was probably due to the HRT.

So I came off it and decided to go for non-drug self-help remedies. I tried aromatherapy, which was very good, and yoga. The relaxation exercises in yoga are helpful, but I also think it is important to make time for yourself. I go to yoga classes and that's a time when I am concentrating on me. I think it helps. At the moment I'm still on propranolol but no HRT and I take vitamin E and evening primrose oil and I manage fine on that. If I get a migraine I take paracetamol or Migravess. I find fizzy tablets very good – even Alka Seltzer helps sometimes. It seems to be working well at the moment but I still haven't managed to lose the weight.

6

Headaches and Other Migraines

Headaches

Tension headaches

This is a very common condition. Approximately eighty per cent of people have experienced a tension headache. The pain is different from migraine in that it is dull, and patients often describe it as the feeling of something pressing down on their heads or like a band being tightened around their heads. The pain can start in the neck and then spread up to the head. Attacks can last all day from morning to night, and although some sufferers find difficulty in sleeping this is not always the case. As the name implies, this type of headache is thought to be due to stress, anxiety or tension. Or it can be part and parcel of depression.

There are several ways of trying to tackle this type of headache. Analgesic tablets don't usually help, according to Dr J. N. Blau in the *Which?* consumer guide *Understanding Headaches and Migraines*, as they are unable to affect or alter someone's mood. Relaxation exercises can help. Yoga, transcendental meditation, aromatherapy, reflexology and so on can help with tension and stress. For more information on these alternative therapies see Chapter 13.

You can also try and find the root cause. Is there something worrying you? Maybe counselling will help. You can look at your lifestyle: maybe you have been taking on too much and are quite anxious about it deep down. Cutting down on the pressure may be all you need to do.

Both tension headaches and migraine can be caused or made worse by using VDUs. This is more fully explained in the A-Z of Migraine Tips and Triggers (see Chapter 15). Hazel, who works as an administrative secretary, has had migraines for nearly thirty years. They come on average about once a month and are menstrually related. Each one usually lasts about twenty-four hours and she takes painkillers and Maxolon to help relieve the pain and sickness respectively.

Hazel

I got my VDU at work about last October. A word processor. It had a white background with black letters on it. We were busy. It was a new piece of machinery I was trying to come to terms with. I got a lot of headaches – one a week and they were lasting three and four days. I hadn't had them like that for about twenty years. Often a headache would start on top of my shoulder and creep up my neck and into the back of my head.

I couldn't think of anything I'd done that was different. Then my yoga teacher said to me, 'You could be allergic to your VDU.' I thought: 'Gosh, yes, maybe she's right.' I stopped using it for a week. I said to the fellas in the office – because they knew I was taking time off work: 'I'm not going to use it for a week, and it helped. Then I heard about these screen filters you can get to cut out the glare and the static. I had one fitted. It was the type that flaps over the top and is stuck on with Velcro. That helped slightly, but I was still getting headaches. Then I came across a company which fitted a mesh right on to the screen. They took the front of the processor off and fitted it on to the screen, and I haven't really had headaches from it since. It cost about £80, but I said to my boss: 'Look, compared with the time you're losing with me lying in bed and not being here, the cost of this is negligible.' It has helped enormously.

The man who fitted it told me I could switch it round to produce a black background with white letters, which causes less glare. That's what I've got now. It's much easier on the eyes. The static and the glare, combined with the fluorescent lights which are on in the office, react on your eyes.

When they install these things they don't tell you. I rang the doctor's surgery because they've recently acquired them up there. They said you should really only work on one for an hour and then have a break and walk around. Also my screen was positioned very much to the right of my typewriter. As a result my head was turning constantly from looking at what I was typing to the screen and so my neck muscles were getting all tight and tense. They said I should really have my screen positioned in front of me so I'm not moving my head all the time during the day and straining those muscles. Now my migraines are back to how they were before – about once a month.

There are many similar filters available from manufacturers of computer accessories.

Trigeminal neuralgia

Because it appears in episodes this kind of headache is often confused with cluster headaches, which are fully described in Chapter 7. Trigeminal neuralgia occurs with equal frequency in men and women, generally in the older age groups. The pain is severe, razor-sharp, or cutting. The symptoms are described by Lee Kudrow in *Migraine: Clinical, Therapeutic, Conceptual and Research Aspects*, edited by J. N. Blau. The slightest contact with the trigger zones on the face can set off the pain, and these zones appear anywhere between the chin and the forehead. Shaving, eating or chewing can trigger an attack, as can even a cold breeze blowing across the face. The attack starts with a sensation of gentle jabbing over the affected area and is followed by a sensation of lightning spasms that last from seconds to minutes.

There is a short gap when the symptoms stop, only to be repeated, and this cycle can occur over and over again for an hour or even longer. The pain, which is excruciating, originates from the trigeminal nerve. These bouts can go on for weeks or months, followed by a remission of months or even years. Anticonvulsant medicines such as carbamazepine, says the Diamond Headache Clinic, can reduce the sensitivity in the face and relieve the intensity of the pain. Unlike cluster headaches, trigeminal neuralgia attacks are unlikely to happen in the middle of the night and awaken the sufferer from sleep.

Chronic daily headaches

Any headache that affects more than 15 days per month is defined by the International Headache Society as Chronic Daily Headache. Some patients may have had migraine for many years and have now transformed into this condition. Other sufferers of CDH may not have had migraine ever before. Some people wake up every day with a headache which sometimes includes migraine symptoms, like nausea and sensitivity to light. However, true migraine does not occur daily.

Chronic Daily Headache can be caused by:

- A head or neck injury.
- Development of an additional headache such as muscle-contraction or tension headaches which can occur daily.
- Overuse of painkillers and/or ergotamine.
- Inadequate management of migraine.

There are different ways of treating this condition. Many sufferers have restricted neck movements which may have been caused by an injury, like whiplash, for instance. Consulting a physiotherapist to improve mobility of the neck can be very beneficial in this situation. You can also do exercises yourself to help loosen your neck muscles. Here are some suggested by the Migraine Action Association. Do each of the following movements twice each day, morning and evening:

- Put your chin on your chest and then slowly move your head backwards so that you are looking at the ceiling and then bring your head slowly back to normal positioning.
- Slowly tilt your head to the side to put first your left ear and then your right ear on to the equivalent shoulder.
- Slowly turn your head so that you are looking as far to the left as possible, then slowly turn it through 180 degrees so that you are looking as far right as possible.

You may also find it helpful to try hot or cold treatments (whichever you find the most comforting) on your neck both before and after the above exercises. You can use a hot water bottle or an ice pack.

Drug treatment can also be helpful in alleviating the symptoms. In the main there are two drugs used. Both were originally developed for other conditions but were found by chance to be effective in patients with headache and are now prescribed for headache alone. Tri-cyclic anti-depressants are one form of treatment; the other medicament that may be used is an antiepileptic drug called Epilim. The latter can present a problem for women if they get pregnant while taking it as it is associated with foetal abnormalities.

Both are available on prescription only and are generally used in much lower doses for CDH than for their other medical purposes. Please see Chapter 11 for more details on drug treatment.

One of the major problems with this type of headache is that sufferers can become dependent on acute headache treatment. As the drugs wear off patients experience a rebound headache and so they take more drugs to counteract that. The trouble is that it is the acute treatments that are fuelling the headache. Treatments reserved for acute migraine therapy should not be taken daily for months or even weeks. What needs to be done in this situation is that the patient has to break the cycle by coming off the drugs. This can, of course, be very difficult and people can experience severe withdrawal symptoms. Some patients may need to be admitted to hospital to be treated.

Other types of migraines

Weekend migraines

It is not uncommon for sufferers to get migraine at weekends or at the start of a holiday. There are several theories for this. It can be a letdown syndrome: the stress and pressures of working all week are put on one side for the time being and you are able to relax – well, you would if you didn't have a migraine! The following explanation is given in the book entitled *Advice from the Diamond Headache Clinic*: 'After a stressful period there may be a letdown which can, in itself, trigger a migraine headache. The arteries may be constricted by prolonged stress, and when the individual is finally able to relax, the blood vessels may dilate, causing the headache.'

On the other hand, people who drink a lot of coffee at work but not when they are relaxing at home, may be suffering from caffeine withdrawal. The A-Z of Migraine Tips and Triggers (see Chapter 15) contains further information on caffeine withdrawal headaches.

Women whose busy time is at the weekend, when the whole family is at home, may suffer migraines at that time because of pressure and stress, or else on a Friday or Saturday morning in anticipation of what is to come. Another possibility is too much sleep. If you are used to getting up early on weekdays and lie in on a Saturday or Sunday, this may cause a migraine. Again, this is more fully explained in the section on Sleep in the A-Z of Migraine Tips and Triggers.

Joan is incapacitated with migraines and headaches. Her bad migraine attacks nearly always come on a Friday in the early hours of the morning. She gets them either weekly or every fortnight.

Joan

I usually get it on a Friday. I get this feeling of being very tired. I yawn a terrific amount. Sometimes it feels as if it's a build up. I'm not a person who can relax much anyway. The doctor says I'm an uptight person. I haven't really got that much to get uptight about. Things do niggle at me. I am a worrier.

I've had migraine since I was twenty-one but I've suffered with bad headaches since I was about five or six. I get a bad headache nearly every day. But with a migraine I get very sick. I go numb all down one side. Normally the pain is on the right side of the head but the complete paralysis is on the left side. I can't even get out to be sick. My husband sort of drags me out. We manage that way. Also the other end. I always have diarrhoea as well. Even if I just have a bad headache I have to go to the loo.

I have Inderal. I take that all the time. A tablet that seems to have helped is amitriptyline – I take one at night. I wake up with the migraine. Straightaway the sickness comes on me. I have to go to the toilet first. After I've had it for about an hour all the left side – the face and mouth down the left side – is paralysed as if I've had a stroke. It's very frightening, but of course I've got used to it now. To start with I was petrified. I thought: 'Whatever is happening to me?'

I am sick through that. Luckily my husband is home all the time because he has retired. When I was younger my children helped me. I have a bowl, because I have to kneel down. I have a prolapsed disc in my back, which doesn't help. He has to hold my back as well while I am retching. It's not just being sick, you're retching and retching. It's ter- rible. Because you're struggling to bring up, it's just yellow-green bile all the time. It's very painful and it makes the headache worse. And then you perhaps get a little bit of easing off just for about five minutes and then – boom – it comes back again. Usually this goes on for a full day. Gradually I can get to sleep, and then the next day I'm washed right out. My mother still gets them and she's seventy-four.

I sit and I moan. It's all I can do. I sit in front of the mirror and I've actually watched myself. It's weird. You're feeling so ill. I sit on the side of the bed and rock from side to side. I don't know what to do with my neck. It's heavy and my head feels as if it's too big. I don't feel I want to talk. I don't want any noise.

My daughter has had it so much with me that it really got her down at one stage. She used to have to stay home from school often if my hus- band had something that took him away. She said it used to nearly make her cry sitting with me.

Abdominal migraine

In this variation the pain is felt not in the head but in the upper abdomen. It is very intense, throbbing and constant and can last as long as eighteen hours. Aura, nausea and vomiting can also be pre- sent. This migraine can be treated with anticonvulsant drugs, says the Diamond Headache Clinic. There is usually a family history of migraine and this type of attack tends to be first seen in childhood. It can progress in later years to migraine with or without aura. Andrew first experienced abdominal migraine when he was around eight years old and they stopped when he was about fourteen. At first the family thought it was appendicitis since the pain was so bad, but abdominal migraine was diagnosed. Andrew suffered about three attacks a year. Now an adult, he still suffers from bad headaches.

Andrew

It would tighten up inside but it didn't last very long. For five or ten minutes it would be very bad, then it would ease off and I'd be OK, but then it would all start up again. It would cramp me up again and the best position was to lie on my side with my knees up to try and relax the stomach. There was no way of stopping it. I had Stemetil suppositories. I even woke up on the morning of my eleventh birthday with an abdominal migraine. I often had constipation as well. If we were out and I got one of these attacks I used to lie on the back seat of the car. I'd be lying there, with a coat over me, trying to use a suppository. Sometimes it was absolute agony and I used to be rolling on the floor with it. The following day I used to feel under. I couldn't do a lot. I'd get cramps in the stomach three or four times the following day.

Rare migraine

So far we have looked at some of the more usual forms of migraine. One of the less common types of this illness is hemiplegic migraine.

Hemiplegic migraine

This rare form of the illness produces paralysis down one side of the body. According to the Diamond Headache Clinic it can occur before, during or after the onset of the headache. The headache itself lasts longer than in most forms of migraine: five to ten days is not uncommon. Vomiting is infrequent and often absent. This information comes from Edwin R. Bickerstaff writing in *Migraine: Clinical, Therapeutic, Conceptual and Research Aspects*, edited by J N. Blau. Between hemiplegic attacks the patient may have attacks of classic or common migraine. In a subsequent attack, the same features and the same degree of weakness develop but on the opposite side of the body; this reversal of sides may alternate in consecutive attacks. There is very often at least one close relative in the family who has identical attacks.

The treatment is the same as for classical migraine but it is important for anyone experiencing this type of attack to see their doctor to exclude all other possibilities. Patients will probably be referred to a neurologist and have a CAT scan (computerized axial tomography) which is a type of X-ray.

Basilar artery migraine

In this kind of migraine, write F. Clifford Rose and M. Gawel in *Migraine – The Facts*, the headache is usually over the back of the head and the symptoms include double vision, giddiness, slurred speech, tinnitus (buzzing in the ears) and sometimes loss of consciousness. The symptoms are due to a diminished blood supply to parts of the brain supplied by the basilar artery, a blood vessel at the base of the brain which goes into spasm to produce an attack.

At one time it was thought to affect mainly adolescent girls, but nowadays it is known to affect people of all ages and both sexes. It is, as in Fiona's case, also known in very young children. However, it is unlikely to start in middle age. Most sufferers have a family history of migraine, but not of basilar artery migraine.

As the attack develops, patients will feel a numbness or tingling in both hands and feet, spreading to the wrists and ankles. The mouth and tongue can also be affected. The initial symptoms can last from ten to forty-five minutes and there then may be a gap of fifteen minutes before the headache starts. This will be severe, throbbing and there is usually nausea and sometimes severe vomiting. This phase of the attack can last for several hours but not usually days. Also known as vertebro-basilar migraine, this is a type of classical migraine which can change to the more usual forms of migraine in later years.

Fiona
(as told by her mother)
Fiona is now six years old. It started when she was eighteen months old. She wanted to lie around. She felt dizzy but she could not really tell me. I thought she wasn't well, but the neurological tests were normal. We found out she had vertebro-basilar migraine when she was about two and a half years old. She gets dizzy and can't walk properly. She is never very keen on bright lights and has sunglasses with her. They help her quite a bit during a bad day. But she's not distressed or in pain.

It usually happens when she wakes first thing in the morning. She can't get out of bed. Or you find her crawling out on to the landing. And she says: 'I've got one of my dizzies.' But you see it goes. If it starts at six in the morning it can be gone by eight that first morning. It gets progressively worse as the days go on until about the sixth day, and then it might be with her all day and after that she'll get progressively better. But the dizziness might be with her over a period of two weeks.

She is a statemented child and has a helper at school. Statemented children are ones who have special needs – who need support either in the educational side of things or on the welfare side. I think she must be the first child who has had to be statemented because of migraine. We were advised to do this before she went to school because these bouts might come and go, and she was not safe at school if she did not have a helper. She feels so insecure that I know she wouldn't step inside the building if she knew she didn't have an adult helper there for her. She likes school.

In with that cycle she also has a behavioural pattern which means that she can be a very difficult child. She gets very high about two weeks before, when she doesn't sleep much. She doesn't sleep much anyway, and she's quite abominable to live with. Speech is a thousand to the dozen. Usually the day before she is incredibly naughty. Then it all comes to light and the next day she is low. Then as she's coming out of it she goes high again. And then she settles down. So you see it is a five-week cycle. In five weeks she's all right for a couple of weeks.

Great Ormond Street Hospital say there's a good chance of her growing out of it by the time she is seven. She'll either grow out of it then or it will become a classical migraine which is more treatable.

I suffer from common migraine. It started in my early twenties. I don't know if there was any family history before that. Usually it's when I've had a lot of disturbed nights. If I can catch it in time I can stop it. I take Migraleve. It often starts during the night. I get a pounding head and I have to sit up. I can't put my head down. The one thing I need is sleep, because it's the lack of that I'm suffering from. But it's the one thing I can't have, because I get this awful migraine in the middle of the night. It's difficult to cope with Fiona as well. I can't be ill in comfort. I just have to cope. At least I'm not sick with it. There are worse.

I had migraines right the way through my pregnancy. I had more migraines during pregnancy than any other time. If I didn't have a migraine I had a headache. I had to have propranolol during pregnancy. I'm not on it now. The migraines aren't bad enough.

Ophthalmoplegic migraine

This uncommon form of migraine is usually first seen in childhood between the ages of four and ten, but it sometimes occurs earlier; it is more predominant in boys than in girls. There will be a family history of migraine, though not necessarily this type of migraine. Pain is the first symptom, in, around and above one eye. It increases in severity as the attack progresses, and can last between two and ten days, according to Edwin R. Bickerstaff in *Migraine: Clinical, Therapeutic, Conceptual and Research Aspects*, edited by J. N. Blau. There can be paralysis in the muscles which surround the eye, causing the eyelid to droop and the pupil to dilate, and double vision may be experienced. Although this disability is temporary and clears up when the attack goes, anyone experiencing these symptoms should see their doctor to exclude the possibility of any other causes.

Retinal migraine

Here, along with a headache, the sufferer endures a repeated blind spot or complete blindness in one eye. The symptoms last for an hour or less. There is also a dull ache behind the eye. This is a rare form of migraine and, again, patients must get medical advice to rule out any other problem.

Other stories

Here are some interesting stories told by migraine sufferers. Robert experienced migraine attacks when he was playing sports. Sports migraines are often a result of low blood sugar, but this doesn't seem to be so in his case.

Robert

One afternoon, when I was twenty-seven, I was playing rugby and started to get blurred vision. I thought I'd been whacked on the head and was suffering from concussion. During the game I seemed to slow down. I went home feeling sick and got a very bad headache which lasted a day.

I had suffered from migraine during puberty. I was thirteen and bringing a Christmas tree back home from the market when I had the first one. I didn't know what it was at the time, but I think I vomited when I got home and I had a throbbing headache. My mother and sister both suffered from migraines. The doctor prescribed Stemetil. In those days I'd get a lot of flashing fights and tunnel vision. Also my mind wouldn't be in conjunction with my brain. I could think clearly and all my words would come out perfectly formed, but they wouldn't come out in the right order in the sentence.

I kept it quiet at school. I couldn't read off the blackboard in one of those attacks. I didn't want to make a fool of myself in class. I'd go home if I felt an attack coming on. I'd get a bad headache and couldn't work anyway.

After puberty it all stopped and I didn't get a migraine until that rugby game. I was very active sports-wise. I played rugby a lot and then there was squash, cricket and training. From that day it built up. Every time I played sport I'd get a migraine. They were different from the ones I had at puberty. I didn't have flashing lights so much, but I did get numbness of the nose and fingertips. And I did get the bad headaches.

I stopped sport altogether. It wasn't worth it. But it was an enjoyable part of my social life and I found it very frustrating watching any sport knowing that I couldn't play. My GP put me on propranolol I only took it before playing sport but, although they took the extreme pain away, they acted as a relaxant. I'm a very competitive chap, but that went and I became very laid-back. The tablets took away the will to win. I'd be playing a game of squash with a couldn't-care-less attitude. Then I was put on Cafergot. That had no effect whatsoever. I was back at square one.

I went to the City of London Migraine Clinic. There was a lady doctor there. She asked various questions. She said that my migraines were obviously linked to physical exercise. She asked 'Do you ever have migraine after sexual intercourse?'

I said: 'No, I don't.'

It took me aback, actually, this lady asking a question like that. But she was quite straight in the face and she asked me again, and I said: 'No, I don't.'

She said: 'You are fortunate, because a lot of people do.'

I thought: 'Thank God for that.' It would hardly be worth doing if I was going to suffer for two days afterwards!

Anyway, she examined me and told me to take two aspirins before playing any sport. Remarkably, it works! I've played rugby all this season and squash twice a week. I take two aspirins before each game and I have no problems now. Maybe if I overdid it I'd get a migraine. But she seems to have done the trick – and I only saw her once!

As well as its analgesic properties, aspirin is also an antiprostaglandin. Prostaglandin is one of the substances which is thought to contribute to the occurrence of migraine.

Rose's story is not so amusing, nor does it have a happy ending. But it does give you a glimpse into what it is like to suffer in silence in childhood.

Rose

I was brought up in Ireland during the Second World War. I lived with my Gran in a lovely fishing village in the west of Kerry. Mum and Dad had found work in West Ham in London. When I was seven I came to live in England. It was quite a change. I had to learn to be a cockney in one day or I'd have got my head bumped in. I've got no memory of migraine in Ireland. That's one of the few bits of my life when I've got no memory of feeling ill or having headaches.

Mum would take us for holidays back to Ireland. The journeys were nightmarish. They lasted twenty-four hours, with a very long time on the train. My head used to be splitting and I used to get sick on the boat. My Mum would get a bit annoyed. She'd give me an aspirin. Of course my family were very tough people. They'd end the journey, as fresh as daisies. They didn't know what a headache or feeling sick was. They'd be as happy as Larry on this awful journey, but it would take me days to feel all right. I remember Sundays when I first came to England. Mum and Dad always had a lie-in and I was meant to look at a book or something until about twelve o'clock. In Ireland I'd have been up and running around in the fresh air. I can remember having splitting headaches then because I'd read and I wouldn't have had any breakfast. They were kind of strict – you weren't meant to help yourself. So that was low blood sugar.

I didn't know them very well. I was a bit scared of my parents. They both worked and I'd come home from school and wait until my Mum got in. She was a nurse. My Dad was a very scary person. When I came over from Ireland I certainly didn't communicate much with them because I was too frightened. They had no idea of kids. They'd had me, and all the time I'd been living with my Gran they'd had in their minds this sort of dream child who would be pretty and clever and know how to tell the time and everything. The actual raw reality that turned up from Ireland was a bit of a disappointment plus I was a terrible weakling. They used to call me 'Weakling'. I probably never told them about the headaches on Sunday mornings, but to this day if I read in the morning my eyes will hurt and that will lead to a headache.

We are a Catholic family. In those days if you were going to take Communion on a Sunday you had to fast from midnight on Saturday. I would have my tea at 5.30 or 6 p.m. on Saturday. Mass would be at 9.30 to 10.30 on Sunday morning. You'd actually get Communion at about 10.15. I can remember feeling very close to death and very inadequate and weak because no one else experienced it. No one but I knew.

There was one occasion when I was about twelve or thirteen when I actually collapsed in church, and that was very frightening. The effect was that you didn't see everything you were looking at – there were bits missing. I thought if I concentrated on the Mass and what the priest was saying I'd cope. But there were lumps of the priest that were black and lumps of the altar had disappeared. I totally flaked out. I can remember feeling very embarrassed and ashamed. But I wasn't with my family. I was with the school, and I can remember a couple of the nuns who took me out being extremely kind. One asked if I got headaches, seeming to know what it was. I was crying and saying I thought I was going blind. But she reassured me and said it was just the headache. I had a few episodes like that until I was about eighteen. But increasingly I had fewer visual problems and more intense pain.

I can remember getting told off by my Mum. I was doing the ironing and she'd bought me a dress, a pink and white candy-striped one. I can remember feeling waves of nausea and just wanting to collapse looking at the dress. The whole thing seemed to be swimming and moving. I said to my Mum: 'I can't do it.' She was very annoyed and thought I'd invented it. So that made me even less likely to tell her if I had a headache. To this day I can't look at anything with narrow stripes. It would all weave and wave and I'd feel giddy. I've had a lot of problems with neon lights. But it's not so bad now that they have got a different rate of flicker and they've got diffusers on them.

Through my pregnancies I'd be very sick and headachey for the first six months – so much so that with the second I was amazed that there was a live baby to come out. It would die down in the last three months, but every migraine I ever missed would come back about three weeks after the birth.

Now I get headaches every day. I always wake up with a bursting head – usually on one side. I quietly potter about and do my jobs. If I'm lucky, it eases off perhaps by teatime. If I'm not, it just gets worse and worse and it'd either be a miserable day and evening or it will go on like that for two or three days. I really can't think back now to a day I woke up feeling all right. But occasionally there will be two or three days that are less bad with just a nagging headache. Those are my best times now.

I've got an extremely nice husband. I think if I'd had someone who was impatient and said: 'Oh God, you haven't got a headache again!' I would probably have thrown the sponge in.

Ruth is twenty-nine years old. She suffers from Down's syndrome.

Ruth
(as told by her father)
It started in 1987. Prior to that she'd had a shunt. They do that to relieve pressure on the brain. They run a line from the head down to the diaphragm so that the pressure can drain off. When she had her first migraine the GP thought it was just a virus. She went a whole twelve months and everything was more or less normal. Then she had this attack again, which he thought might possibly be migraine, and after that she was having them about every three weeks quite regularly. They lasted for about twelve hours. There was much vomiting and what have you, but after twelve hours it was OK.

We had all sorts of checks done and everything else was OK, so it all boiled down to migraine. Then they put her on Sanomigran. That seemed to be helping. She even went ten weeks without one. Then when she had one it was pretty bad. Instead of being twelve hours it went to twenty-four hours and it was pretty severe too.

When it starts off she goes very quiet. She says her tummy feels funny and her head feels funny and she can see lights. Then the vomiting starts. That comes every half-hour – heavy vomiting. That goes on for a full twenty-four hours. She might sleep for an hour. It's the headache that really seems to destroy her. It reduces her to tears. She can't stand light. She has to be in a darkened room. She can't stand much sound, either. She can't take anything by mouth at all during the whole of that twenty-four hours – even a sip of water can make her retch. Now I've got her on propranolol only.

She's not severely disabled. She can get about and do things. Her speech is restricted. But she is bright enough. She can assess what's going on. She can follow the television. She can communicate during the migraine. She lets us know what's hurting. Sometimes she will get a violent shaking, almost like an epileptic fit. She's had an EEG just to check on that, but there's no epilepsy involved. She almost leaps out of bed and her whole body shakes. She lost her mother last year, which accentuates it a lot.

Laura gets migraines roughly three times a year. She started getting them when she went on the contraceptive pill and continued to get attacks even when she came off it. Now, some fifteen years later she gets them so badly that in a recent attack she thought she was going to die and contemplated going into her children's bedroom while they were asleep to kiss them goodbye.

Laura

When it first starts it's always my right hand. Even though I don't appear to be looking at it my hand seems to be growing. I can't really take my right eye off my hand and I'll even walk with my hand behind my back trying not to look at it. It just seems to appear enlarged all the time. From there, again in my right eye I get like a fountain of light streaming out of my eye and then flashing lights until my vision becomes blurry. I can't focus. If I'm walking towards the wall I'm not in a straight fine. I'm out of alignment.

I then lose speech and my hand goes numb. I think at the time I could actually stick a knife in it and I wouldn't feel a thing. This goes on for about an hour and a half. Then the headache comes and that's terrible. I really feel as if my head is going to explode. For a couple of days afterwards I can't move it. It feels as if it has really been punched – I can't turn round quickly or anything like that.

It was the middle of the night and I was in such a lot of pain I thought my head was going to explode. I thought I was going to die. It sounds daft now, but at the time I really did think that. I nearly woke up my children to give them a kiss as I really thought I was going to have a brain haemorrhage and would not be there in the morning. They were aged eleven and eight then.

The next four days I felt as if I wasn't there. I was on another planet. I felt miles away from my body. The doctor said it could have been like a mild stroke it was so severe.

Claire gives a very interesting and lucid description of her aura and symptoms.

Claire

I've had them, with all the peculiar emanations, since I was a child. I used to smell burning, and the cracks on the plaster and the walls from the bombing used to walk. I can't remember visual disturbances during the day, but I can remember the smells and seeing spiders that weren't there and this thing about the hands feeling huge, and I know now it was the same feeling I got as in Alice in Wonderland. Exactly as Lewis Carroll described it – the growing and the shrinking – and I can remember lying in bed at night and feeling myself shrinking down to the size of a pea. I never said anything to anyone because it was fanciful, and I'd get told off for being fanciful.

Both my parents suffered from really dreadful headaches.

My mother had the vomiting. Dad had them with double vision and migraine spots. And I'll never forget one night he was sitting in a chair and he told us afterwards he had this huge spot move across his vision and he just ignored it, and the next thing Mum and I were climbing up the tables because it was the biggest spider in the world. It was real! He used to get that type of visual disturbance. Mum would complain of squiggles. With her it was terrible vomiting that she suffered from.

I didn't suffer from the vomiting – I just used to get these odd disturbances. And then of course when puberty set in I started to get the headaches. But nobody said anything. I think at that stage it was probably not to frighten me, because I had watched all the family – and when I say all the family I'm talking about my father, my mother, her brother, her father. It wasn't until I was twenty-two and married that the doctor said: 'What you've got here is migraine.' I didn't tell the doctor about the body disturbances, because he was a rather old gruff man who just dealt with the headaches and didn't seem terribly interested in the aura.

I still get the hand and the shrinking, and this precedes a headache. Very, very occasionally I get what I call battlements. I see the up-and-down shape that you get on the top of a castle in the top left-hand corner of my field of vision. But when I get all this it's a good warning and I take tablets: Migraleve, and I'm also getting a great deal of help from a drug called Froben which is a non-steroid anti-inflammatory one.

I can feel each individual tooth throbbing. They feel huge and they all hurt. My whole body feels huge and gross and I can feel each individual part of it huge. That feeling goes along with a weird disembodiment. I can't think straight. My head feels completely scrambled. I have to lie down. I feel as if I've been punched in the face, and I occasionally get a nose bleed. The skin is sore, and then it's the temple and then the nails in the eyes and then into the joint of the jaw and down the jaw and all the teeth, and that can last a good twenty-four hours. The body feeling lasts a couple of hours. The head only pounds if I move. If I can keep still it's OK. It's as though my brain is turned to jelly and red-hot, and every movement makes the jelly quiver and every quiver is painful. The next day my skin is actually sore as if it's been burnt. My whole head is sore. It hurts to comb my hair and I'm usually feeling nauseated from the drugs. My husband says I go grey. The soreness is in the head where the pain was.

Nowadays the getting larger and smaller doesn't frighten me because I know what it is. Getting smaller was frightening, because there was that feeling of falling as well and it makes you feel a bit sick. That's happened to me during the day. I'd be sitting here at my desk and I've felt as though I was falling through the bottom of the chair. Lewis Carroll had it to a tee.

I try very hard not to live in fear of it. But I avoid discos. I make sure I eat regularly. I take food when I travel, I also avoid late nights. It's difficult, because my husband is an Aberdonian and they're a sociable crew. It makes it difficult for me in family gatherings.

7

Cluster Headaches

Symptoms

This very rare condition is predominantly a male disorder which affects less than 0.1 per cent of the population. About five men to every woman suffer from cluster headaches. The condition used to be known as migrainous neuralgia but now it is not thought to be migraine at all. However, sometimes cluster headaches are diagnosed as migraine and vice versa.

They are called clusters because they come in bouts. The patient may have an attack every day for a period of, on average, six to twelve weeks, but then he or she will be completely symptom-free for a few months, a year or more. Remarkably, many patients have their period of clusters at about the same time every year; it is even more common for sufferers to experience an attack at the same time every day. Many patients suffer more than one attack a day and some sufferers can also have chronic cluster headaches with no respite for several years.

This type of headache is extremely painful. One of the characteristics is that patients are unable to stay still. They pace up and down and rock backwards and forwards; many bang their heads against the wall and press down on the affected eye with their hands. Sufferers have said that they become so frenzied during an attack that they throw things around the room. Mark gives a good description of an attack in his story. The headache is almost always one-sided and always the same side. Very occasionally it will affect the opposite side in a different cluster. The pain will have a stabbing, burning or piercing quality, and it is centred around the eye. Other symptoms include a stuffy or runny nose, together with a red and watery eye and drooping eyelid on the affected side.

The attack usually comes on suddenly, with little or no warning, and often awakes the sufferer during the night. Most cluster headaches last around forty-five minutes but they can last as little as fifteen minutes or, in rare cases, as long as three hours. The frequency and intensity of the headache are often at their lowest at the beginning and sometimes towards the end of the period of clusters. Other people experience a 'storm' of clusters just before the end of the bout.

Alcohol is known to trigger an attack, but only during a cluster period. The attack will come on about half an hour after alcohol has been consumed. Nitroglycerine, which is used in the treatment of angina, can also trigger an attack, while smoking can make it more severe. However, giving up smoking will not cure the condition.

Treatment

It is not known, writes J. N. Blau in *Understanding Headaches and Migraines*, whether the pain comes from local blood vessels dilating or from the nerves supplying these vessels. Treatment is usually concerned with trying to prevent an attack, which is difficult since virtually no warning is given. Ergotamine tartrate can be very effective in the treatment of cluster headaches. Dr Blau writes:

> One effective way of taking ergotamine is in suppository form. If the attacks are happening at night, the suppository should be inserted before going to bed. If attacks occur during the day, a suppository should be inserted in the morning. After a few nights of freedom, the dosage can usually be reduced by cutting off a portion of the suppository so that only three-quarters, two-thirds and eventually one-half is being used. As with any drug the minimum effective dose should be taken.

Another way of using ergotamine is through an aerosol inhaler called a Medihaler. One of the plus points of using ergotamine for cluster headaches is that it does not usually have adverse side effects when used for a short period of time like six to eight weeks, which is the average length of a cluster bout.

Other drugs used to treat cluster headaches are methysergide, lithium, prednisolone and pizotifen. All of these are described in more detail in Chapter 11.

A different and often effective way of aborting a cluster headache is inhaling oxygen. Again, Dr Blau explains:

> Inhaling oxygen from a cylinder at a rate of seven litres per minute, using a firm plastic mask, can abort attacks within five to ten minutes. This method works for about six out of ten patients. The oxygen cylinder should be kept by the bedside so that as attacks begin the oxygen can be inhaled. Having the correct mask is important. A large oxygen cylinder is needed, because the oxygen flow rate must be seven litres a minute (small cylinders manage only four litres a minute). General practitioners working

within the National Health Service are able to prescribe oxygen for cluster headaches.

Tony talks about the use of oxygen for cluster headaches in his story. It is thought that oxygen causes the blood vessels to constrict if it is inhaled at the beginning of a headache.

Here is a very explicit first-hand account of cluster headache attacks. Mark is a salesman with three children. Despite the fact that he has suffered badly with cluster headaches for over eleven years – one bout lasted for eighteen months – he has been very successful in his work, winning trophies and prizes for salesmanship. Mark is also very sporty: he used to play a lot of football, and is a blue sash at kung-fu.

Mark

They call it a suicide headache. It's the best way to describe it. I've never felt pain like it. I do martial arts. I fight every week. It's the worst pain I've ever known. It really is excruciating and there is no relief. It affects behind my eye, my nose, my teeth, my neck, shoulder, and all down the left-hand side of my face. The pain – people say it's like a sword going in your eye and being waggled about. I suppose that's quite a good description, but it's a throbbing pain as well.

It's always on the left-hand side of my face. It can last as long as an hour and a half, but it seems to me that it builds up until it reaches a peak. Let's say an average attack would last for an hour: from that first five minutes it will build, so thirty minutes into the attack I'm literally banging my head against the wall. It really is agonizing. You can't talk. Your eyes water. Your nose runs. You've really got to pace up and down and try and get rid of the damn thing. I like to get on my own somewhere, but not on my own in a dark room. I have to try and fight it. I've had migraines in the past, where you feel really rough with a headache, lie down and hopefully go to sleep and get rid of it. This isn't anything like that. You need to pace up and down. When I'm at home I go to the bedroom, I'll come downstairs, I'll go back up again into the bathroom, and I'd be moving all the time, trying to fight the pain.

My wife and kids would see me rolling around in agony. I do try and get up to the bedroom and keep it to myself, but everybody knows what's going on and they can't help but know. You do tend to moan a bit as well. They say that's to help relieve the pain, and it does seem to help. I've tried not to let it affect us as a family, but obviously it does. I always used to have it round about Christmas. It used to ruin Christmas because I'd spend part of it upstairs. Once I'd got rid of the headache I'd come back down again and be part of the family like normal.

If I'm on the road, I obviously have to pull in. If I'm on a motorway, that's the biggest dread. I pull over to the side because I can't drive. I can't do anything. I have to get through it and carry on again. Obviously if I'm on a motorway I can't, but on a normal road I get out and try to go for a walk. It's a bit difficult because you're having a job to see and, not only that, it's a bit embarrassing because people are looking at you. So sometimes I just sit in the car, but I'm moving all the time, trying to rub my head or shoulder. You do need to move constantly.

The last ten minutes, as I start to go out of it, it's quite a relief really. It's like little electric shocks – I can feel it changing. The electric shocks are in the temple, or in the ear, or down the side of the neck. They're not drastically painful. It's quite pleasant when I get those, because I know it's going. Gradually it will taper off.

I've tried about forty different things. Painkillers don't touch me. The only thing that touched it was when I had five attacks in one day, lasting about an hour each. I called the doctor in the end and he gave me morphine. That worked. I've tried acupuncture, chiropractic and feverfew – none of them were any use. I've been on Deseril, Sanomigran, ergotamine and Tegretol – without success. The one trigger that really sets it off is alcohol.

I was treated for sinus. I went to the doctor and he gave me various sprays, He even sent me to a specialist. I went to have sinus X-rays because my nose was always blocked during an attack. The specialist thought there was something wrong although the X-ray was clear. He'd never heard of cluster headaches.

Mark eventually landed up at the Princess Margaret Migraine Clinic at Charing Cross Hospital. After a CAT scan and other tests he has been put on a calcium channel blocker (see Chapter 11) which seems to be helping.

Lisa used to be a schoolteacher. One day the children she was teaching decided to play a prank on her. She was using an old fashioned self-standing blackboard and they booby-trapped it. As she stood in front of it, it came crashing down on her, knocking her unconscious. She was in hospital for a week and the migraine came on soon afterwards. Several years later the clusters started. Now she has both migraines and clusters, but the migraines are more manageable. Until last year she was spending two months of each year in hospital because of the cluster headaches. She has two young sons, and that meant missing out on a large chunk of their childhood.

Lisa

They come around January or February every year and they last for twelve weeks. When they first start they usually come at night. They wake me up. My left eye goes very red, very bloodshot. My nose blocks up and then it starts running at the same time. It is a tremendous pain which goes through the eye on the left side of the head. The pain is not a headache. Not like migraine where you want to lie down. It's like when you are in labour and you don't know where to put your bottom on the couch. You don't know where to put your head for comfort. At home I tend to walk about. I'll sit down, put my head between my knees. This lasts for about an hour if it is untreated. The longest on one occasion was two hours.

At the beginning stages of the cluster I will probably get one a night. But in the middle stages I can have them every two hours throughout the night. I have three weeks at the beginning and three weeks at the end, so the middle phase can take about six weeks. I'm hardly getting any sleep anyway, because I'm only just getting back to sleep when it starts again. I'm absolutely shattered. My eyes get very badly inflamed. I can't drive. I'm not an awful lot of use anyway. I get so exhausted.

They started four years ago. I tried all the things you can try: ergotamine, methysergide, lithium. I don't react well to drugs. I tried steroids and I went down to six stone. Eventually it came down to just treating the pain with pethidine.

The trouble is it's such a long period of time. They started me off on a dose of 50ml but towards the end I was getting 300ml for an attack. It's a heck of a lot of pethidine. Oxygen works at the beginning and at the end of the phase. No painkilling tablet is of any use because it doesn't get into the system fast enough. I have to have an injection.

During the first three weeks I only have the oxygen, and when I get to the stage of having an attack every two hours I'm admitted to hospital. I've been in for eight weeks in one go. In hospital I have the pethidine injections and the oxygen. This year they taught me how to do the pethidine injections myself. They gave me an orange and an ampoule of water to practise on, and I injected myself with water when I didn't have a headache. It's very painful and it's difficult to control your hand while you put the injection in. I inject in the thigh. I'm quite slim and that's the worst thing, finding a place to put it in. My legs looked beautiful at the end.

But they let me come out once I could do the injections. The trouble is that you have to keep increasing the dose because you get tolerant to it. Then as the headache starts to get less you cut down on the pethidine, but your body starts craving the drug and I could see that I could very easily have injected the pethidine when I didn't need it. I asked my

*father to look after the ampoules for me. When I went into dreadful
withdrawal symptoms they took me back into hospital to help me come
off it. You feel on edge. Your body feels as if it's crawling. All I want to
do is rub my arms and legs. Walk up and down. I'm a musician. I used
to go and play the piano. I just had to take my mind off it. My hands
were shaking and I'd get the wrong note but it was just something to dis-
tract me.*

*The previous year I was in hospital during withdrawal and I was
hallucinating then. I don't remember a lot of it, but my husband said I
was talking about gremlins. They sedated me quite heavily last year.
They didn't do that this year.*

*I sometimes get cross. My youngest wouldn't come near for a bit
when I came out of hospital. He was afraid to get too close in case I went
away again. We are quite a close-knit family and we do a lot of things
together.*

*Fortunately my neurologist suffered from clusters himself and he's
very sympathetic, but each time I go into hospital there are young doctors I've never seen before even though the nurses don't change. It takes
all the time I am there before the young doctors really understand what
they are dealing with. In fact the nurses drag them in and say: 'You've
got to see her during an attack.' But the doctors say: 'Oh well, a
headache is a headache.'*

*I have to plan ahead. If I'm buying birthday cards I'll buy them for
the whole year and I'll have them all written out and leave lists for my
husband so all he has to do is put them in the post. With two boys, when
you're back in charge at home there's no time for putting your feet up.
I've been told by my consultant that his clusters went at fifty – so I've got
another eleven years. There's always the chance that they might come
up with something else.*

George, a computer programmer, has had three main attacks of cluster headaches in the space of about seven years. In the last one he
experienced a dull pain behind his eyes which lasted continuously
for the cluster period, which was six weeks. Added to this were the
attacks of severe pain which he would get daily.

George

*One morning I woke up completely cross-eyed. A few nights before I had
had a really bad headache and I took some tablets for migraine. It had
said on the packet that one in a thousand people suffer from loss of
co-ordination. I thought to myself – 'This is pretty severe lack of co-
ordination!' This stayed with me for a month or so. The pain came and
went. I decided to wear a patch over one eye, and just concentrate on*

one eye and I could see just one of everything. I was in the first year of a degree and I was doing my mock exams. I took my three exams with a patch over one eye, and that weekend the pain disappeared and I was able to take the other three exams normally.

That was the first attack. I've had two more since then. The last one was the worst. The eye trouble started up again just in the left eye. Five days later both eyes hurt and my mouth hurt if I ate. My acne got worse. It was a dull pain at the back of the eye all the time. I like pop music a lot. Other people might find it upsetting, but it suits me. I found that by putting the music on it was like bringing something back. It was something I could grab on to. So that's what I would do. I know some people say that noise is really bad, but I found it relaxing.

I went to the Princess Margaret Migraine Clinic and saw one of the doctors, who diagnosed it straightaway as cluster headaches. I had the really bad pain and I started to feel really numb as well. I was put on steroids – prednisolone 5ml. I took twelve for two days, ten for two days, eight for two days, six for two days, four for four days and two for eight days. When I was on twelve the pain went completely. But by the second day of eight the pain was back, and if anything I think it was worse. Every morning I would wake up with a shooting pain in the eye. I would see it was four o'clock exactly – not five minutes either side. I'd hold my head, and if the pain was really bad I'd get hold of my hand and push it against my eye. I felt a bit nauseous. Also my tongue was numb during the cluster.

I was actually at work when I was taking these steroids. At one stage when I was down to about six I was in a conference room for about half an hour and I wasn't able to work – I wasn't able to do anything, the pain was so bad. I was due for my next steroid in half an hour and I was in the conference with my head in my hands. Before that people used to call me 'Mr Cool' because I was wearing my sunglasses all the time. After a while they realized it must be serious.

My boss took me into a small room and it was a fully fledged meeting. They said they thought it would be best if I took time off while I was on the steroids because it had been noticed that I was hyperactive around the office. I am one of these people who likes to joke around a bit more than most, though I get the work done. But I think it was a lot worse than normal because of the steroids. I was disruptive, they said. So I took a fortnight off work.

At the end when the steroids were finished I saw another doctor at the clinic, and they put me on Epilim which is normally associated with epilepsy. As it was towards the end of the attack, I don't know whether it was time or the Epilim that had worked.

Tony has had cluster headaches for twelve years. Attacks can last from two to five months with about nine months free in between. He was on ergotamine for eight years but has since had an angioplasty (heart operation) and cannot take the drug now.

Tony

I was taking Medihaler a couple of hours beforehand once I knew the cycle of it. Then nine times out of ten the pain wouldn't come. Now I can't take the ergotamine I don't know what I'm going to do. The ergotamine is very bad for the heart. I took it every day during the cluster period. I never had withdrawal symptoms.

A typical attack is a runny nose and pain over my left eye and down the left side of my face through to the back of the neck. The pain can vary from the back of my neck through to the eye. It usually starts in the eye. I always know when it is coming because my eyes dilate quite a lot. The attack lasts a minimum of two to three hours, with a maximum of five to six. The only thing I know that does trigger it off is alcohol. If I drink alcohol, within about ten or fifteen minutes it comes on. But only during a cluster period.

Sometimes the Medihaler didn't work. Luckily when it didn't I could take pure oxygen for about fifteen minutes and it would clear the headache virtually immediately. And it wouldn't return until the next day. So I always carry an oxygen cylinder around in the car, and I also have one at home. It's the size of a briefcase. But I can't take it on a plane. It can't be pressurized, so you have to empty it and then get it filled up again when you're abroad. Now when I'm on holiday I always check with the hotel that they carry oxygen – a lot of continental hotels do. I can either fill up my own cylinder or use theirs.

Another problem with the oxygen is that nobody knows whether it should be on a prescription or not, or how much to charge for it. My GP couldn't understand how much oxygen you get through having a cluster. He thought I was going over the top, but I wasn't. I find I go through two lots of oxygen cylinders in a week. I had to get a letter from the specialist saying that it was quite all right to use this kind of quantity, otherwise the doctor would have refused to give me a prescription. To get oxygen abroad is very easy.

Before I got medication it affected my working fife. Once I got a pain I had to go to bed with a Valium. Then when I got on to Cafergot I'd go to bed with a Cafergot suppository and a Valium and that was it – I was out for about three hours during the working day.

I can sometimes feel a pain coming when I'm in the car. I pull into a lay-by or whatever and just go into the back of the car and take the oxygen cylinder out and open it up and use it. People look at me as if I am absolutely mad. The police once were very suspicious when they stopped me and saw this oxygen cylinder there. They asked me what it was for, and I said it was for medical reasons. They thought I was stark raving mad. So I said: 'I'm actually using it as a blowtorch for a safe job, and then they left me alone!'

GPs don't understand clusters. They think migraines and clusters are the same, which they are not. I have got to the stage of literally banging my head against the wall just to relieve the pain with another kind of pain. I also try pressing on the pressure points, and sometimes it does make the pain go away.

8

Migraine in Children

Symptoms

When you consider that nearly one-third of migraine sufferers get their first attack before the age of ten and that there are 6 million migraine patients in the UK, you can see how many children experience the illness at one time or another. Although in many ways their symptoms are very similar to those of adult migraine, the difficulty with children is in communication, especially when they are very young. Childhood migraine is often linked to travel sickness. Most children suffer from migraine without aura, and the headache is usually throbbing and at the front of the head. Often they wake up with a headache. There may be nausea and vomiting. Very often they have tummy ache. This may be in addition to the headache, or it may be there on its own. The latter is an abdominal migraine, and a graphic description of it was given by Andrew in Chapter 6.

It is important to try and get a clear picture of the symptoms, both for your own peace of mind and so that you can give the doctor as full a description as possible. If your little one is clutching his head, maybe (but not necessarily) to one side, is off his food, wants to be quiet, is listless and yawning, it may be migraine. If he looks pale, is irritable and perhaps staggering about, these are other symptoms. Some children do get a visual disturbance: in Chapter 2 Jane described hers. But Jane is an older child; a younger one may say 'My eyes have gone funny' or 'I can see fireworks' or 'squiggles' or 'wormy things'.

In Chapter 6 Claire says that, as a child, she never told her parents she used to feel herself getting larger or smaller because she was afraid of being thought 'fanciful'. And both her parents were migraine sufferers! So do take the 'squiggles' and the 'worms' seriously. Don't automatically assume that the child is winding you up – especially if there is already someone in the family who suffers from migraine. Visual disturbances can be as frightening for children as they are for adults. Discuss migraine with your child, and explain that the visual symptoms are just part and parcel of it. By the way, children migraineurs are very often light-sensitive, so that's another warning sign to look out for. On the plus side is the fact that children's attacks usually last for a much shorter time than adults.

It is worth going to the doctor even if, at the back of your mind, you are convinced that your child is suffering from migraine. Headaches accompanied by fever must be reported to your doctor, and check out the stomach ache as well to be on the safe side.

As with adults, migraine in children is often mistaken for sinusitis. The most common symptoms of sinusitis are runny nose, persistent cough and recurrent ear infection. The best way to diagnose sinusitis is by X-ray.

Self-help treatment

Dr J. N. Blau, an eminent authority on migraine, says he can cure many of his child migraine patients in one session and without resorting to any drugs whatsoever. His method is quite simple – he gets them to eat breakfast.

So we're back to talking about blood sugar. Children can be devils at breakfast-time – to get them to eat anything is a nightmare. But eating breakfast is important for all children, and for the migraine sufferer it is a must. Take this scenario: little Michael has a cup of hot chocolate before going to bed at nine o'clock. He will not have breakfast next morning, but by eleven o'clock at school he is ravenous so he buys himself a nice chocolate snack. School dinner is 'yuk', so he moves it around the plate instead of eating it. (Or if there is a school shop he buys himself some chips, another bar of chocolate and a can of Coke.) By the time he gets home at four o'clock – surprise, surprise, he has a headache. Not only has the intake of sugary food along with the fasting brought his blood sugar level down to an all-time low, but he will probably have played sports and had a rough and tumble with his mates, and this use of energy will have precipitated a further drop in his blood sugar levels.

Breakfast is a battle you really must win. Cereal or toast is fine, and neither takes long to eat. Fruit juice or tea are equally easy breakfast-time drinks. If you can get him to take a piece of fruit or a bread roll with ham, tuna, salad or whatever to eat as a snack during the day, so much the better.

Migraine in children may be triggered by the same foods that trigger adults. Chapter 9 discusses food triggers. But do bear in mind that it is important to ensure that your child eats regularly and has a varied diet. If your child is food sensitive remember that if you are giving your child a painkiller in liquid form they contain additives to help them look and taste nice and also to extend their shelf life.

These can be sugars, other sweeteners, preservatives, flavourings and colourings. All these may cause allergic reactions.

Remember that when a child is suffering an attack he or she is feeling very unwell, in pain and probably frightened as well. They will want to be in a quiet, dark place and they may or may not want to be alone. Jane in Chapter 2 does, while Amanda – who, incidentally, is my daughter and tells her story in this chapter – does not. She usually suffers an hour of intense pain and likes to have someone with her then. So put your child to bed, if he or she is ready for it, but skip the bath and teeth-brushing routine and stay with them at least for a while if you can, or keep popping in to reassure them that they haven't been forgotten.

Medical treatment

If you can catch the attack quickly enough, a simple painkiller like paracetamol – in tablet or liquid form – may be all that is required. A fizzy form of paracetamol often works better. Stay with your child while he or she takes the medicine. You would be amazed at the number of children who flush the pills down the loo or hide them and then claim that they don't work! Children under the age of twelve should not be given aspirin.

Since it is so important to get the painkiller into the system as quickly as possible, it is worth having a chat to your child's teacher. If the child can feel it is 'safe' to tell the teacher when he or she thinks an attack is coming, and get immediate treatment, a great deal of unnecessary anguish can be saved. Also, if there are visual symptoms involved, tell the teacher about them and give her or him the gist of the medical explanation. All you need say is that they are caused by the blood vessels narrowing and that the headache comes when the vessels dilate. The point is that your child needs to be taken seriously – not laughed at.

Although many of the drugs used for children are the same as those used for adult migraine patients, they are used in different dosages. A child's body weight is less, and in very young children the liver and kidneys are not fully developed. All this has to be taken into account when prescribing. So don't be tempted to give your child a little less of what you take – get medical advice first.

Propranolol or Sanomigran are occasionally given to children as preventative medicine. Most doctors try not to give children daily drugs. It is not a good idea to start children relying on tablets. As a rule children who are on daily medication for frequent headaches should come off treatment after a short time.

Amanda is twelve years old. She suffers with migraines without aura and experiences a lot of nausea although she is not sick. She has not as yet started her periods and there is no particular pattern to the timing of her attacks. There don't seem to be any food triggers.

Amanda

We were on holiday in France, living in a tent. One day my parents said we were going to drive into Spain. It was a long way and we had to drive round and round a very long and windy road down some mountains [the Pyrenees]. I started to feel sick. Dad kept saying: 'Look at the amazing view.' But I felt sick. When we got to Spain Mum looked strange as she got out of the car. She said she felt dizzy. I thought: 'Oh no, we're both going to get migraines. Poor old Dad.' But we had this brilliant meal and Mum said she felt better and so did I.

Then we went to a museum and saw some paintings, which was really boring, and then we did some shopping and it was time to go back. I thought it wouldn't be so bad going back, because it's usually quicker and I thought I could go to sleep in the car.

As we started to go round the mountains I started to feel sick again and then came the head. It was throbbing really badly. We had some Panadol [paracetamol] in the car but we had forgotten to bring anything to drink, so I couldn't take them. Anyway, Mum said I would probably be sick if I did take them. We couldn't turn the car round because the road was too narrow and windy, so we kept going.

My head was hurting so much and it felt so hot that I felt it had turned into a volcano which was bursting and all the lava was running down the side of my face, burning it, and running into my eye and burning that. And we kept going round and round up this mountain. I wanted to cry but I couldn't. Everybody kept very quiet in the car hoping I'd go to sleep, but I couldn't. I kept thinking my head was going to burst. I really thought it would. It was so frightening. I kept my eyes shut because the sun was still shining and it really hurt my eyes.

When we got to a straight road it felt a bit better. I didn't feel quite so sick. When we got to the tent Mum started looking for the Paramax but my sister, who is eighteen, and very bossy, said I should have a Panadol immediately. Mum said I should try and sleep it off in the tent and she and Dad would be outside. But I didn't want to be on my own, even though I knew they could hear me if I wanted anything. The sun had gone down and I sat outside feeling dreadful.

A little bit later one of my friends came. She was going back to England the next day and she wanted to take a photo of me with the others. My Mum said she didn't think I was up to it. But I thought: 'If I don't go they'll forget me.' So I said I'd be all right and I went to my

*friend's tent. We had Coke and crisps and we took photos and I realized
that my migraine had gone.*

Ryan first started having migraines when he was six years old. The
first came a few days after he had had an accident in which fractured
his skull. He is now eleven and according to his mum has been
through hell with the migraines.

Ryan
(as told by his mother)
*It was a swing in our garden. He ran from our back door and dived
head first on to it and missed it and went straight through and bashed
his head as he went down. He broke a bone over his right temple. It was
a straightforward fracture. He did it at 8.30 in the morning. I checked
him through and said: 'We must let your school know you've had a head
bang this morning.' He was OK until about one o'clock, and then they
rang me and said he had started vomiting. I think then I knew he had
actually fractured his skull.*

*He had his accident on a Friday and he spent the night in hospital.
He had a terrible eight hours while he was vomiting and was in quite
a lot of stress. It seemed to pass and he came home on the Saturday. He
had all the symptoms again on the following Tuesday. He had a
headache and was sick. He was that bad they readmitted him. Looking
back, I think that was his first migraine.*

*When he started with them I just went to the GP. I also got lots of
books out I tried to find all the answers myself. Then things became
really bad and Ryan was having about two a week where he was being
sick with them. They were just leaving him like a dish rag. He would
wake up in the night crying and holding his head and vomiting. It
would last about an hour. He said he used to feel as if his whole head
was open and he had a raging fire in it and big people were hammering into the middle of his head.*

*I used to get him to do deep breathing and I invented this little relax-
ation garden which, if anything, I think helped the vomiting. We went
down these steps with beautiful trees and we always sat on this one seat.
And there was a duck pond. In our minds we just created a little garden. He actually made a model of a migraine garden with fresh flowers
and won a prize for it. It helped him through a bad period. Now –
maybe it's because he's older – when he has a bad one he just wants to
be left alone.*

*What worries me is that now when he has a migraine he finds that
going to bed and lying down doesn't actually help him. Before, when he
went to sleep he would still wake up with a headache, but it was a*

headache he could cope with.

One particular night he came back from Scouts and he literally fell through the door and his little temple was actually pulsating as if his head was going to burst. You could see his temple bulging. He was a terrible colour. I'd seen it before but I'd never seen it that bad. And he just flung himself at me.

I got so I couldn't cope with it any longer. I needed some help. My husband and I were worried sick about him. We went to the school doctor and he said we should take him to the hospital. He had a scan and it was fine. The paediatrician said they were migraines. He monitored him. He was given Paramax, which was useful provided Ryan took them at the onset of an attack.

I went through a very bad period where I tried to suppress him but, as my husband says, he's a child and he has to live life as a child.

I work and he knows he can ring me. But he doesn't. He'll last out all day and then collapse in a heap on the settee when he comes home.

The migraines have lessened to one every six weeks, but we've had good runs like this before and all of a sudden they've come back with a vengeance. But after four years I am coping much better than I've ever done because I feel I've looked in every flipping book and I've tried so hard to help him. I now know that there is nothing further I can do – just be there for him really.

Eighteen-year-old Zoe suffered a bad patch of migraine headaches when she was about ten. She saw an allergist, who put her on a low-fat diet which excluded all dairy products. The migraines lessened and soon after that went completely, but they came back two years ago when she was taking her GCSEs. She had also given up the diet.

Zoe

I get an attack round about period time. The last one I had was really bad. I had just had a bad cold. I woke up in the middle of the night with this terrible pain in my eye. It felt as if someone had got a poker and put it through my eye, on to the pillow and through the mattress in my bed. I felt as if I was pinned to the bed with this poker going through my eye. I couldn't move. I couldn't speak. I wanted to shout for help but I couldn't. It seemed to go on all night.

It was a bit better in the morning and I was able to take some paracetamol. The pain gradually subsided but I felt washed out all day.

I don't get migraines that often. They don't come every month and they are not usually that bad. I suppose if they were I would have to think about going back on my diet. It was so boring. The low fat wasn't so bad, but doing without milk in any shape or form is a real killer socially. Everything's got milk powder or whey powder in it. You can't keep examining packages, and when you go round to friends' houses you can't exactly drive their parents mad. I mean, suppose your boyfriend's mother cooks something really nice, you can't exactly ask her if it's got milk or butter in it, can you? It's almost bound to have.

Mind you, if I kept waking up in the middle of the night with a poker in my eye I suppose I would have to think it out again. But there's no guarantee that if I did the diet it would work again this time.

9

Migraine and Food

The main foods thought to trigger migraines in some people are chocolate, cheese, alcohol and citrus fruits; then to a lesser extent pork, bananas, onions, fish and wheat flour. Many people also report having fewer migraine attacks once they give up caffeine. Certain people are sensitive to monosodium glutamate (MSG food additive 621) which is used in large quantities in Chinese food (soya sauce in particular) and as a flavour enhancer for many of the food items we use every day – stock cubes, for instance, often contain MSG as do soups, sauces, pies and cooked meat products.

A migraine attack will not occur straight after the particular food trigger is consumed, but later on in the digestive process, when the food has entered the liver and is being processed by the enzymes. Doctors now think it is here that the chemical action can go awry in some people, causing the wrong breakdown of food and releasing substances that can open wide the blood vessels of the brain. Known as vasodilating amines, these substances occur in many foods, but the two most common ones are tyramine, which is present in many cheeses, and phenylethylamine, found in chocolate. Dark chocolate is more suspect than milk chocolate. Some cheeses – cottage cheese, quark, Philadelphia and curd cheese – have no detectable traces of tyramine. At the other end of the scale are blue cheeses which have a very high tyramine content. Synephrine, a vasoactive amine, is present in citrus fruit. And alcohol is itself a vasoactive substance.

Tracking down the culprit(s)

Many migraine sufferers drive themselves mad on the diet front. One woman complained that she barely ate anything for fear of a migraine attack. You can't live like that. But bear in mind that, if you do manage to track down a food that triggers your migraine, you are one of the lucky ones: you can give it up. But you have to be organized and determined to do it well. Try jotting down everything you eat or drink over the next three to four months, along with the time of day when you consumed it. This may sound laborious, but it's not as difficult as it sounds if you keep a diary in the kitchen. Those of you who have been to Weight Watchers will be well used to the routine, and at least I'm not asking you to weigh your food!

See if any particular food or foods always crop up thirty-six hours or less before a migraine. If there is more than one, work by elimination. If you suspect that cheese, chocolate and bananas may be triggers, cut out all three. Then if there is no improvement in your migraines, you know you are barking up the wrong tree. If there is, it may be just one of the three questionable foods, two of them or all three. Reintroduce the foods one at a time to see if you can isolate the culprit.

When tracking down possible food sensitivities you must exclude the suspect ingredient from your diet entirely. If you are excluding milk, for instance, it is not just a question of doing without it in tea and coffee. Milk appears in various forms in all sorts of packaged and prepared foods. Cheese is out, of course, as are butter and all other dairy products. With citrus fruits, marmalade is an obvious food to drop, but remember also to scan the contents of tinned and packaged foods in case oranges, lemons or limes have been used for flavouring. This kind of meticulous investigation of everything you eat is essential – it may be a bind, but then so is migraine. Remember also that a food that triggers a migraine during menstrually sensitive times may be perfectly all right, in limited quantities, at other times. Try it. The better you know your body and its reactions, the more control you have over your migraines.

If the daily jottings are too much for you, you may like to keep a retrospective chart. The post-migraine period, when you can remember just what it was like, may be the best time to put pen to paper. The best chart is probably one that you devise for yourself, taking into account your lifestyle. Here are some things to consider when making your chart.

For many migraine sufferers it takes more than one trigger to start a migraine. For example it could be perfectly safe to eat some cheese on a normal, peaceful day or when your period is not due BUT combine cheese with a stressful day at the wrong time of the month and you can be in migraine trouble.

To be really useful your chart should include the following details:

DURING THE 24 HOURS BEFORE THE ATTACK

a) Date of attack, time of month, time of migraine attack
b) Extra excitement, shock or stress
c) Unusually busy day, or end of busy time
d) Any travelling

e) Insomnia, sleeping late, a lie-in
f) Missed meals or start of diet
g) A record of everything you ate or drank in the 24 hours before your migraine started and the approximate times you ate.

Don't study the completed charts until you have several to compare with each other. You will need to keep records like this for 3 or 4 attacks before a pattern can begin to show up. By ignoring the references to menstruation, children, men and older women will find this chart idea equally useful.

Doctors, Tests and Clinics

Doctors

A market research company recently researched doctors' attitudes to migraine. Here are some of their findings:

1 GPs have a low level of concern with migraine, as they do not consider it a dangerous condition.
2 Very few are aware of any new product.
3 Even if other causes are suspected, such as PMT or menopause or stress-related problems, doctors treat the symptoms rather than look for a root to the problem and treat that.
4 GPs are unaware of the current level of effective therapies – they only know that patients do not revisit their surgeries and hence assume that the product has worked.

Very little in the above findings is going to be news to migraine patients. We also know that many doctors and some neurologists do not find migraine an interesting condition. This often puts sufferers off going to the doctor. We believe that he or she has got more important things to do than worry about our migraines. This cannot be true. The average GP does eight to ten surgeries a week, seeing roughly thirty-five to forty-five patients a day, according to E. Ian Adam writing in *Migraine: Clinical, Therapeutic, Conceptual and Research Aspects*, edited by J. N. Blau. If the majority of these patients did not have run-of-the-mill and uninteresting conditions the nation's health would be in a sorry state.

The other point to bear in mind is that it is the illness that the GP may find uninteresting – not you. If you are business-like and informed about your symptoms the doctor will sit up, take note and relate to you as an intelligent and interesting person. If you can give a clear description of your symptoms, and know the kind of questions your doctor is going to ask, you will be treated with interest and respect. This in turn will make you feel good about yourself and more positive about finding a solution to your migraines. So here are some guidelines:

1. Book a double appointment

On average the doctor allows six to eight minutes per patient. This may not be enough to cover the ground. So if your GP runs an appointments system, book a double appointment with the receptionist to give yourself and your doctor more time.

2. Look good

Take a little bit of trouble with your appearance. This is not to try and make the doctor fancy you, but if you look good you will feel good, and you will then be more in control and feel less intimidated.

3. Make a list

Write down everything that happens during the course of an attack: how it starts, what sort of times (morning, evening, middle of the night, weekends) and so on. Include any warning signs or aura you may get. Take this description with you to the surgery, and then you won't panic about trying to remember everything.

4. Answer the questions

There is nothing quite like knowing what you are going to be asked to enable you to give clear and detailed answers. Dr J. N. Blau is a neurologist who is very interested in migraines. In his book: *Understanding Headaches and Migraine* published by the Consumers' Association he lists the questions that doctors are likely to ask. Here are some of them.

- When did the headaches start?
- How long do they last?
- How often do they occur?
- What brings them on?
- What precedes them?
- Where do the headaches start?
- Does the pain move during an attack?
- How severe is it?
- Does anything make the headache worse? (for example, coughing, straining or bending down)?
- What makes them better?
- Are they associated with anything else (such as nausea or a dislike of bright lights)?
- Does any other member of your family have headaches?
- What sort of an effect do headaches have on your life?
- What have you already tried for the headaches and what effect did this have?

- Why have you decided to seek help now?

Obviously the doctor will not necessarily ask all these questions, and he or she may ask one or two not mentioned. But if you know the answers to those listed above you will certainly be able to give a detailed picture of your migraines. If you have made a note of the pattern of your attacks and any triggers you will have very little difficulty in answering the questions about severity of pain, where it occurs, what precedes it and what accompanies it. But there are one or two questions which may be worth a closer look. For instance:

When did the headaches start?

Did they start in childhood, puberty, with the onset of menstruation, pregnancy, the birth of a child, menopause, a particularly stressful time, change of environment and so on? It is worth thinking about this, because it can help the doctor gauge the cause of your attacks. If it is hormonal it may require a different form of treatment than if environmental conditions or stress were the trigger.

Why have you decided to seek help now?

If you have been suffering with migraines for years and have been treating them yourself you will be in the majority of sufferers. According to the survey 70 per cent of patients never, or no longer, consult their GP, although 77 per cent feel that their work or daily activities are impaired to some degree or they cannot function at all. Only 7 per cent of migraine sufferers regularly consult their GP. So, why now? Have the migraines got worse? Are they different? Are they bothering you more now than they did before, or have you finally had enough and want to do something about them? If they have got worse or are different, try and make as detailed a comparison as you can. Maybe you no longer experience a visual aura but get a very much more severe headache. Maybe you only experience the aura and are frightened by it. Maybe there is more vomiting or diarrhoea. Maybe the attacks last longer or are more frequent. If the change is more in your attitude than in the migraines themselves, ask yourself the following question.

What do you expect from the treatment?

You may want a cure but you know by now that, as far as migraine is concerned, it is unlikely. Good management is the next best thing. So what would this be for you? There are basically two forms of management: those that seek to prevent the migraine from occurring, and those that minimize the severity of the attack. Of course, taking prophylactic (preventative) treatment very often also reduces the severity of those attacks that do occur. The trouble is that most prophylactic treatment entails taking the drug every day for some months, and drugs can have side-effects.

Obviously, if you get weekly migraines that last a couple of days you are going to want something that at least cuts down their frequency, and this may well come in the shape of one of the preventative drugs. Many migraineurs' lives have been changed by taking a daily drug. If you are put on a preventative drug, ask the doctor:

- What the side-effects could be.
- Are there any contra-indications? In other words, are there conditions or situations where you shouldn't be taking the drug. For instance, diabetics, asthmatics and bronchitis sufferers are unlikely to be prescribed propranolol since the drug can cause breathing difficulties and affects the body's response to low blood sugar. (The doctor will have a note of your medical history, and that will be taken into consideration before prescribing, but there may be other, less obvious doubts that you want to clear up.)
- How long you are likely to be on the drug.
- When you should return for a check-up. The doctor needs to know how you are getting on with the treatment. So if he suggests you return in a month's time, make the appointment before you leave the surgery.
- Be very clear about the dosage. Write it down so that you don't panic when you get home: 'Did he say one a day or one three times a day?' Sometimes the dosage is indicated on the label but it may just say: 'As directed by the physician' or another nebulous phrase which leaves you totally at sea.

If your attacks come once a month or every three months even less often, you are far less likely to be looking for preventative treatment, bearing in mind the side-effects. What you want is something that handles the attack by either minimizing its severity or aborting it at an early stage. It may be that all you need is meto-clopramide with a painkiller; or you may require a much stronger painkiller. Alternatively, if your attacks are infrequent and your warning signs clear, ergotamine taken at the onset may abort them. Another drug which can successfully stop an attack for some sufferers is the new drug Imigran. Again, ask the doctor about:

- Side effects
- Dosage
- Contra-indications

• Follow-up appointment

If the treatment the doctor prescribes does not work, GO BACK. Don't give up. Most of us don't get everything right the first time we try – why should your doctor be different? Give him or her a fair chance. If after a few visits you have experienced no real improvement, ask to be referred to a neurologist or a migraine clinic.

Migraine clinics

The main advantage of attending a migraine clinic is that they are very well clued up on current thinking and treatment. The City of London Migraine Clinic was established in 1971. In its first four years the clinic treated two thousand patients during an attack, while six-thousand people attended between attacks. The clinic works as a medical charity in conjunction with St Bartholomew's Hospital to provide treatment and advice to patients referred by their GP, hospital or company doctor. A referral letter is always required except for non-UK residents. However, it also offers emergency treatment for patients in an acute, untreated, normal-type attack of migraine which has started that day. Patients from any part of the British Isles can be seen as long as they are eligible for NHS treatment. Patients from abroad can be seen privately, as can any patients who are covered by private medical insurance. It is financially supported by the Migraine Action Association as well as other benefactors.

The Princess Margaret Migraine Clinic, which is part of Charing Cross Hospital, in London will treat patients on the National Health Service while they are suffering acute attacks. It also receives financial help from the Migraine Action Association.

So what happens? If you visit the clinic during an attack, and if the attack has been untreated and started that day, you will be shown into a darkened room and treated by a doctor or senior nurse there and then. If you attend between attacks you will have a consultation with a doctor who is interested in migraines and knows a good deal about them. This is, in fact, the most helpful treatment. It is so much easier to discuss your condition with a doctor when you are migraine-free. Not only are you in a better state to understand the advice given, but with a clear head, you can concentrate on telling your side of the story.

The clinics do not only exist to treat patients; they also do valuable research into the whys and wherefores of migraine and effective drug treatment. For instance, the efficacy of combining the antinausea drug metoclopramide with aspirin was first discovered at the

City of London Migraine Clinic. The same clinic took part in trials researching into the effectiveness of feverfew on migraine patients, and more recently the effects of the new Glaxo drug Sumatriptan.

In addition to these two London clinics, many neurological departments in NHS hospitals see migraine patients. Sad to say, at the time of writing many of these clinics (including the London ones) are under threat of closure through lack of funding. As government spending in this area becomes increasingly restricted, the clinics turn more and more to charities such as the Migraine Action Association and other interested parties.

Tests

Although the cause of headaches is very seldom anything sinister, doctors like to play safe and get any reasonable doubts out of the way before or while treating for migraine. This is usually done by careful physical examination but if the doctor suggests you have an X-ray it is not because he thinks you have a brain tumour but because he has to make absolutely sure that there isn't any underlying abnormality. Sometimes these tests are performed for research purposes. Here are some of the tests you may be asked to have:

Computerized Tomography (CAT or CT scan)

In this X-ray, many views are taken of the brain. The machine moves in a way which enables it to focus on one thin slice of the brain at a time. This kind of precise and detailed screening picks up abscesses, tumours and other malformations in the brain. The patient is asked to lie very still under the scanner, and the procedure can last for about twenty minutes. There are no side-effects.

Electrocardiogram (ECG) and Electroencephalogram (EEG)

The more common ECG is used to measure the electrical activity of the heart, as abnormalities can be picked up from the wave patterns produced. The electrical activity of the brain can also be recorded by placing small metal electrodes on the scalp and measuring the activity using the EEG. Normal patterns of electrical activity in the brain include what is known as alpha rhythm when the eyes are closed; it becomes slower when the eyes are open. Patients on tranquillizers produce fast rhythms, while brain malfunctions or tumours produce slower waves.

Lumbar puncture

In this test a sample of cerebro-spinal fluid (CSF) is removed for analysis. This is done to rule out the possibility of diseases like meningitis or subarachnoid haemorrhage. In the latter the headache is severe, at the back of the head, and comes on suddenly. It is due to a burst blood vessel on the surface of the brain. The test is usually done under local anaesthetic. The patient lies on his or her side and a fine needle is introduced into the lower back to remove a small quantity of fluid.

Arteriography

This is not performed as often as a CAT scan, because the procedure can be uncomfortable and it is therefore usually done under general anaesthetic. Dye is injected into the neck arteries which supply the brain. X-rays are then taken, which will show up any abnormalities.

11

Drug Therapy

Choosing the treatment

Most people who manage their migraines usually do so with the aid of drug therapy. For some this will mean no more than taking a simple painkiller as and when an attack occurs, while for others it may entail taking, on a daily basis, a drug to try to prevent attacks. Obviously the best drug therapy is the one that achieves the desired effect with the minimum amount of drug intake. Trial and error and a patient doctor are the necessary ingredients for this recipe.

But the question that most of us ask ourselves at some time is this: which end we should tackle the problem from? Do we go for prophylactic treatment that has us swallowing pills every day or do we treat each attack as it comes? For many people the solution is obvious. If you get infrequent migraines there is little point in taking daily medication, better to concentrate on getting the best treatment to curtail the severity and length of the attack. Patients who get migraines that put them out of action on a weekly or fortnightly basis are going to be interested in preventative treatment. But what about those of us who live in the grey area where, for example, we get a monthly migraine which lasts two or three days – do we go for prevention or what?

It is very much a personal matter but one useful measuring rod is the extent to which it affects your life. Some people say that although they write off two days every month, they live life to the full the rest of the time. There seems little point in prophylactic therapy in this situation. But if that two days means that you cannot hold down a job or that the threat of a migraine looms so large that you curtail your activities and live in constant fear, preventative therapy could change your life. Whichever you decide to go for, you will need medical help and advice; in Chapter 10 we discussed how you can make the best of the sessions with your doctor.

Drug naming and taking

You may have wondered why the same drug seems to go under two names. Some people refer to pizotifen while others will call the same drug Sanomigran. In fact all drugs in general use have three names. The first one is given by the Nomenclature Committee of the British Pharmacopoeia Commission which consists of doctors, pharmacologists, pharmacists and chemists. This is the official medical name and it is a generic term for the basic active substance of the drug. The second is a brand name given by the manufacturer of the drug. Different manufacturers will give different brand names to a drug which has the same basic active substance. In addition to which, this basic substance may be combined with other substances to produce a slightly different medication which will have yet another name.

Pizotifen is the generic name for Sanomigran. You will notice that Sanomigran is much easier to remember and pronounce than pizotifen. Brand names are produced with the user in mind and usually have the benefit of marketing skills. Combination drugs often describe what they are. Cafergot, for instance is a combination of caffeine and ergotamine – again instantly memorable and descriptive.

The third name is the chemical and technical one. To those outside the medical profession it is an incomprehensible mixture of numbers and letters and happily need not concern us in this book.

Described below are some of the drugs most commonly taken for migraine – but please don't take this as a substitute for talking to your doctor about any drugs he or she may prescribe for you. As far as taking drugs are concerned it is important to take them early at the start of an attack. Take them with a large glass of some form of non-alcoholic liquid (water is a good one!). And take them standing up or sitting if possible. If you take them lying down or dry they can get stuck in your oesophagus which is not only likely to delay the action of the drug but it won't do a lot for your oesophagus! Tablets taken in soluble form are more quickly absorbed into the bloodstream but if you have non-soluble tablets you could try taking them with a sweet fizzy drink.

Much of the information on drugs in this chapter and indeed throughout this book has come from the *British Medical Association's Guide to Medicine and Drugs*. This is an extremely informative and easy to read reference book which you should find in the reference section of your public library.

Painkillers

There are many painkillers (also known as analgesics) available for the treatment of migraine and many patients find that these, sometimes taken together with anti-sickness tablets help minimise the severity of attacks. Many simple analgesics can be bought over-the-counter and it is a question of trial and error to find the one that suits you best. Although painkillers are most commonly taken by mouth and swallowed, they are also available for placing under the tongue (sublingual) or in suppository form.

Do bear in mind that taking too many analgesics over a period of time can cause problems and lead to a condition known as Chronic Daily Headache. See Chapter 6 for details.

Drugs taken by mouth are absorbed into the bloodstream through the walls of the intestine. Drugs taken on an empty stomach, for example before meals, are likely to act more quickly than drugs taken when the stomach is full. Sublingual tablets which are placed under the tongue and not swallowed are absorbed quickly into the bloodstream through the blood vessels in the lining of the mouth. Painkillers in suppository form are given to patients who experience severe vomiting and therefore cannot absorb the drug orally.

It is worth remembering that taking too many analgesics can actually cause headaches. Taking any acute headache treatment **regularly** on more than two or three days per week can be associated with increased frequency of headaches.

Aspirin

Although it is often effective when taken at the very beginning of an attack before pain actually starts, aspirin is not suitable for everybody. Children under the age of 12 should not be given it and sufferers whose migraine includes nausea and vomiting might be advised to avoid it because of the possibility of gastric irritation.

Patients with a present or past peptic ulcer should not take aspirin, nor should those who are aspirin-sensitive. Asthmatic patients are especially liable to such sensitivity. It is estimated that 4 per cent of asthmatic patients are affected. Symptoms of aspirin sensitivity include wheezing, bronchoconstriction and skin rashes. Cross-sensitivity between aspirin and ibuprofen has also been reported. The interaction between aspirin and anti-coagulants is well-known and the two drugs should only be taken together under medical supervision.

Aspirin is widely available in 75mg tablets for angina or heart attack patients and sometimes for migraine prevention. To treat an acute attack 600mg is considered to be the therapeutic dose. So it is advisable to buy packs of 300 mg tablets. Enteric coated aspirin tablets are easier to swallow but can take longer to work. The soluble form is best.

Paracetamol

This is effective for some patients and has the benefit of being free from gastro-intestinal side-effects. However, patients should bear in mind that the maximum adult dose of paracetamol-containing products is 4g daily, i.e., eight 500mg tablets. Exceeding this dose is dangerous as it can cause liver failure.

A dose of less than 1 gram of paracetamol is unlikely to be effective in treating a migraine attack. Many products contain sub-therapeutic doses of paracetamol as concern about its overdose potential becomes more widespread. Purchasing a sub-therapeutic dose is a waste of money.

Paracetamol is one of the safest drugs available. However, fears of overdose have resulted in recent legislation prohibiting the sale of paracetamol in quantities in excess of 100; larger quantities now require a doctor's prescription. Purchasing paracetamol in super-market quantities of 16 tablets is an expensive process but requests for 50 or more tablets at a pharmacy may result in interrogation by a pharmacist. It is therefore advisable to make yourself known to your local pharmacy as a migraine sufferer. This will enable the pharmacist to advise you on the most suitable treatment for you as an individual and facilitate the purchase of larger quantities of paracetamol if required.

People who are concerned about the possibility of overdose may purchase a product which also contains the antidote (methionine) such as Paradote. Such products are naturally more expensive and the patient runs the risk of taking two medications when only one is necessary. However the evidence is that these products are safe and can be used with confidence if concern of overdose is an issue. Pregnant women should stick to paracetamol alone as the safety of the combination in pregnancy is not known.

Non steroidal anti-inflammatory (NSAIDs)

These affect the production of pain-producing substances in the body. They also reduce stiffness and inflammation particularly in joints, bones and muscles and are usually prescribed for arthritic and rheumatic conditions. However some migraine sufferers find them helpful where other painkillers have failed. Ibuprofen is available without prescription. Asthmatics are probably best advised to avoid ibuprofen because of the possibility of sensitivity, as already mentioned. NSAIDs should also be avoided by patients on anti-coagulants or anyone who has or has had a peptic ulcer.

Diclofenac (brand name Voltarol) is a commonly used NSAID for migraine which is available on prescription.

A new drug on the market is Clotam which is a non-steroidal anti-inflammatory analgesic containing the active ingredient tolfenamic acid.

Combined analgesic products

There are dozens of mixed analgesic products containing aspirin, paracetamol or codeine. From a pharmacological viewpoint, a dose of at least 15mg codeine is required for an analgesic effect. Constipation and nausea are possible side effects with codeine. Since it also shuts down the gut, which is already a problem with migraine, codeine is best avoided for attack treatment. Some of the proprietary combinations are available in dispersible or soluble forms which will act quickly and may therefore offer an advantage.

Caffeine is often included in some of these combination analgesics for its mood lifting effect. The point to consider here is what you want the pills to do for you. If you want to ease the pain so that you can carry on with your activities a combination that includes caffeine is not a bad idea. However, if the only way out for you is to try and sleep it off, avoid an analgesic combination that includes caffeine. Remember too that caffeine is a stomach irritant so if nausea and vomiting are involved, steer clear of it. Solpadeine contains codeine, paracetamol and caffeine. Syndol contains codeine, paracetamol, caffeine and doxylamine (a muscle relaxant). Midrid contains paracetamol and isometheptene which constricts the blood vessels.

Analgesics combined with anti-emetics

Migraleve combines the antihistamine buclizine, which has anti-sickness properties, with paracetamol and codeine. The pink tablets contain all three ingredients and are designed to be taken early in the migraine attack. The yellow tablets contain paracetamol and codeine. Migralift is a very similar medicament. These products are worth a try where nausea and vomiting is associated with a migraine headache.

Some products containing antihistamine can cause drowsiness so check the label before you take them.

Since the digestive system is so much part and parcel of migraine, there are drugs which kill pain and keep the stomach moving.

Migravess for instance contains aspirin and metoclopramide. Paramax is a combination of paracetamol and metoclopramide. Metoclopramide has a direct action on the gastrointestinal tract. It is used where there is a need to encourage normal propulsion of food through the stomach and intestine. It is a powerful anti-emetic and is most commonly used to treat nausea and vomiting. In other words, it keeps the stomach moving which helps the pain-killing part of the drug to be absorbed. Metoclopramide causes drowsiness and can also cause constipation or diarrhoea. It should not be given to children as they are more prone to side-effects.

A new combination is Domperamol which brings together domperidone (10mg) and paracetamol (500mg). Both constituents have been in use for many years, paracetamol as a pain killer and domperidone as an anti-emetic with similar action to metoclopramide but with fewer side effects. Relief of symptoms is usually experienced within two hours. You can repeat the dose every four hours but you should not take any more than eight tablets in 24 hours.

Like all treatments taken just for migraine attacks, domperamol is not recommended for continuous use and should not be taken as a preventative treatment. It also is not recommended for children under the age of twelve, pregnant women or anyone who is known to be allergic to its ingredients. The drug should not be taken in conjunction with other products that contain paracetamol, domperidone or metoclopramide. It is advisable to tell your doctor if you are on other medication, particularly, antimuscarinics or blood thinning drugs such as warfarin, bromocriptine, cholestryamine and opiates.

Narcotic analgesics

These are very strong painkillers which are related to opium and can be addictive. They act directly on several sites in the central nervous system that are involved in pain and they block the transmission of pain signals. These drugs can cloud consciousness and prevent clear thought. They can also produce nausea and vomiting, constipation, drowsiness and they can depress breathing. When taken in overdose, narcotics can induce a deep coma and cause breathing difficulties which can be fatal. These drugs are not readily prescribed as they can also produce feelings of euphoria which can lead to mis-use and addiction. However, they can be helpful in treating severe pain provided they are only taken for a short time. Many doctors feel that narcotic analgesics are not ever necessary for the treatment of migraine as the short and long term side-effects outweigh any benefit from these drugs.

If you want to know about the joys of coming off pethidine read Lisa's story in Chapter 7. Pethidine is sometimes given as an injection to sufferers undergoing a particularly severe migraine attack, but it is also available on prescription. Another drug in this category is pentazocine (brand name Fortral). This drug is similar in action and use to morphine. It is a short-acting drug which is less likely to cause breathing difficulties and drowsiness than other narcotic drugs. But it can increase blood pressure and it can also sometimes cause confusion and hallucinations.

Anti-sickness

These are of paramount importance in the treatment of migraine. Metoclopramide (brand name Maxolon) is one of the most useful since it keeps the stomach moving, making it empty faster so that the medicaments will be passed into the small intestine and be absorbed more quickly. According to F. Clifford Rose and M. Gawel in *Migraine: The Facts*, levels of aspirin in the blood stream have been found to be twice as high after metoclopramide has been given. Maxolon should be taken 15 minutes before other drugs to help absorption. It can cause drowsiness.

Domperidone is an effective anti-sickness drug which has an advantage over other anti-emetics in that it does not usually cause drowsiness. Like Maxolon, it increases stomach motility and is also available as a suppository. The brand names are Evoxin and Motilium.

Prochlorperazine (brand name Stemetil) is another anti-sickness drug widely prescribed for migraine and often taken in conjunction with painkillers. It is different from Maxolon, say F. Clifford Rose and M. Gawel in *Migraine: The Facts*, in that it has a powerful anti-nausea effect but it does not affect the motility of the stomach. Stemetil is also available in suppository form. It can cause drowsiness and dizziness.

Ergotamine

This is a drug that is used mainly to treat severe but infrequent attacks. It is now less widely prescribed because of potential side-effects and the possibility of overuse problems. Ergotamine comes from a mould that grows on rye. The mould, called ergot, contains a mixture of substances one of which is ergotamine. The first people to come across the dark side of the ergot were medieval Europeans whose flour for making bread was produced from rye. The trouble was that the flour was milled from mouldy rye; and as a result victims developed a severe rash and discoloration of the fingers and toes and, in extreme cases, their limbs developed gangrene and dropped off. The disease was known colloquially as 'St Anthony's Fire'.

Sufferers would take themselves off on a pilgrimage to the shrine of St Anthony in Italy. It was a journey that took several months and you might have expected them to arrive there limbless – but quite the reverse: they were often cured before they got there. In those days it was no doubt put down to Divine intervention, but today we have a more down-to-earth explanation. Ergot constricts the blood vessels. Large doses taken over a period of time would cut off the blood supply to the extremities – hence the gangrene and loss of limbs in very severe cases. However, those who made the journey were probably not acutely infected and as they moved away from the area of the mouldy rye they started eating bread that was not contaminated. As the ergot came out of their systems they started to get better and even cured.

It is this action of constricting the blood vessels that makes ergotamine so useful to migraine sufferers. Migraine, particularly with aura, is thought to be caused by the blood vessels first constricting and then swelling and dilating. At the constriction stage many sufferers get the aura or warning symptoms. At the dilation stage they get the pain. Ergotamine, taken at the aura or warning stage can pre-empt the pain by preventing the blood vessels from swelling. So ergotamine is not a painkiller. Patients who do not know this often keep taking ergotamine throughout the attack hoping it will lessen the pain. As a result they often wind up, ironically, with an ergotamine-induced headache. If it doesn't work at the beginning of an attack, switch to something else.

Ergotamine headaches are often mistaken for migraine because they are accompanied by nausea, but these headaches are dull, nagging ones rather than the throbbing sensation of migraine. They are continuous, often worse in the morning, prompting the sufferer to take more ergotamine for the 'daily' migraines. However, true migraine does not occur daily. Coming off ergotamine can make the headache worse until the system is cleared of the drug. Patients suffering from ergotamine overdose may have to be taken into hospital when they are coming off the drug. Ergotamine is related to the drug lysergic acid (LSD) and can cause hallucinations.

The point to know is that people vary in their tolerance to ergotamine. The drug stays in the body for a long time which is why periods of rest from ergotamine are very important. As a general rule you should not take more than one or two doses of ergotamine in any one week and always start with half a tablet or half a suppository as it may be enough.

If you are taking ergotamine several times a week or on a daily basis and you have a headache virtually every day, you could well be suffering from ergotamine-induced headaches. You should see your doctor to get medical help to come off this drug. It is no good taking a painkiller or migraine drug to get rid of an ergotamine-induced headache. Only more ergotamine will work but that, of course, will push you further up the spiral.

Side-effects of ergotamine taken in recommended doses include nausea, vomiting, shaking, trembling, cold hands and feet, muscle cramps, abdominal pain and a feeling of weakness. Overdosing can lead to addiction, chronic headaches, damaged arteries, seizures and hallucinations. Thankfully gangrene is a very rare side-effect these days but it does rarely happen. Often a toe will feel dead. Obviously if this happens stop taking the drug immediately and see your doctor straight away. Ergotamine was at one time used to speed up uterine contractions in labour and ergot derivatives are still used in obstetrics. Anyone suffering from heart disease, artery disease and strokes should not take this drug.

If taken early in an attack, ergotamine can work for some sufferers. Patients with cluster headaches are often successfully treated with this drug. Migraine sufferers who get very severe attacks but perhaps less than three or four times a year could discover a very powerful ally in ergotamine. Patients who have infrequent attacks of classical migraine might find this drug useful because they have a clear warning of an impending attack and can use the drug to abort it. Sufferers from common migraine without aura who are well clued into their warning systems may also find it useful for cutting out the pain stage. However, anyone suffering from migraines more often than once a month should think very carefully before starting on this form of treatment. If your doctor or specialist prescribes it, discuss the possible side-effects. Also it may be worth arranging some regular medical monitoring of how often you take it to ensure that the amount you take doesn't creep up unnoticed.

Ergotamine is available in several forms. The most common is tablets but very little is absorbed. You can also get it in an inhaler similar to asthma inhalers and as suppositories which are more likely to be effective. These are useful for people whose migraines are accompanied by severe vomiting or who suffer gastric stasis early on in the attack. With an inhaler or suppository the medicine gets through. This drug is often combined with other substances for a variety of reasons. Cafergot, for instance, is a mixture of ergota-

mine and caffeine. Because caffeine has a similar effect as ergotamine in narrowing the blood vessels, mixing the two in a tablet, suppository or other form of medicament, makes the drug quick-acting
and efficient. In some compounds ergotamine is added to drugs
which act against nausea and vomiting – Migril is one. Lingraine is a
brand name for ergotamine tartrate.

A short story

Before we leave the subject of ergotamine, here's a story with a
happy ending. The Migraine Action Association received a long, sad
letter from a young man living in India. He wrote to say that his
father was at the end of his tether and threatening to commit suicide.
His migraines, which had always been bad, were now continuous; in
addition, he was suffering from stomach pains, nausea, aching
muscles and was feeling constantly weak and ill. The young man said
that his father was desperate and he was afraid that he would make
good his threats and take his own life.

The symptoms rang a familiar bell at the Association's head-
quarters. They wrote back to India saying that the father might not
be suffering from increasingly frequent migraines but from overdosing on ergotamine. They suggested that he sought medical advice on
those grounds, obtained help in coming off the ergotamine and
should be put on a different kind of therapy for his migraine attacks.
The Association heard nothing for some months and then they
received a phone call from the daughter. She was visiting England
and rang to say that her father had taken the advice and the family
were delighted with the result. He was off ergotamine, on a different
form of treatment and although he still suffered migraine attacks, he
was able to handle them. Best of all, he was leading a full and happy
life between attacks!

5-HT agonists

This group of drugs has been developed from research into serotonin, a chemical found in the brain which is released into the blood
stream. Serotonin influences the size of the blood vessels making
them either dilate or constrict – depending on the initial size of the
blood vessels. It is thought that at the first stage of the migraine,
serotonin causes the blood vessels to constrict, allowing less blood
and less oxygen into the blood stream. This produces some of the
neurological symptoms of the aura or other migraine attack warn-
ings. Then the blood vessels go from being constricted to being
dilated. At this stage the warning ends and the pain begins.

Although ergotamine has effects on the serotonin system, more specific drugs have been developed which have fewer side-effects.

Imigran (sumatriptan) was the first drug of this type to be launched by Glaxo Wellcome in the early 1990s. It is not a preventative treatment. You take it when the attack occurs.

It is available in three different forms. The tablets are 50mg or 100mg and are swallowed whole with water soon after the onset of an attack. If symptoms are relieved for a while but the migraine comes back, you can take another dose but you must not exceed 300 mg in 24 hours.

Imigran injections are faster acting than the tablets because the drug gets into the bloodstream more quickly. These injections are available in pre-filled syringes with auto injector so that patients can inject themselves soon after the onset of an attack. They are not difficult to use. If the migraine returns another dose can be taken after an interval of at least one hour. You should not take any more than two 12mg injections in 24 hours.

The injection is also licensed to treat cluster headaches.

The nasal spray comes in a pump applicator which contains one 20mg dose. You use it by blocking one nostril and squirting the drug into the other. You then breathe out through the mouth. The nasal spray is also faster acting than the tablets. Patients who experience vomiting early on in their migraine attack or who need rapid resolution of symptoms, may find the injection or nasal spray more effective than the tablets.

If your migraine does not respond to the first dose of Imigran, in whichever form you take it, it is not advisable to take a second dose for the same attack.

Zomig (zolmitriptan) is the one of the latest of the 5-HT therapies and is produced by Zeneca. It comes in tablet form and the normal dose is one 2.5mg yellow tablet. It should be taken at the start of an attack and you should experience relief within one to two hours. If this does not happen a second dose can be taken after two hours. If you find that you need two doses before you can get an attack under control, it may be best, in a subsequent migraine attack, to take one 5mg dose at the start. You can take a further tablet if symptoms return after initial relief. No more than 15mg should be taken in any 24 hour period.

Zolmitriptan is different to sumatriptan in that it has a dual action. It prevents the constriction of the blood vessels and it also works centrally on the part of the brain stem known as the trigeminal nucleus. It is thought that pain originates in this location of the brain.

Naramig (naratriptan) arrived on the market in the same year (1997) as zolmitriptan. It is produced by GlaxoWellcome and, like zolmitriptan, it works centrally. The pale green tablet contains 2.5mg of naratriptan hydrochloride and should be swallowed whole with water. One tablet is the recommended dose and this should be taken at the start of **the headache phase** of the attack. Relief should be experienced within four hours. If the first tablet does not have any effect it is unlikely that further doses will help. However, if relief is experienced but the symptoms return, you can take another tablet after an interval of not less than four hours. No more than two tablets should be taken in any 24-hour period. Naratriptan is claimed to have fewer side effects than sumatriptan with less chance of the migraine recurring.

None of the 5-HT agonists are recommended for people over the age of 65 or for women who are pregnant or breast-feeding. Neither sumatriptan nor naratriptan are licensed for children under the age of 18. Zolmitriptan has been used for adolescents (which is usually considered to be children over the age of 12) with some success, although it is not licensed for this purpose.

This range of products is not suitable for rare forms of migraine such as vertebro-basilar migraine or familial hemiplegic migraine.

They may not be suitable for anyone with kidney problems and should not be taken by patients with uncontrolled high blood pressure, heart disease or circulation problems. They must not be taken in conjunction with ergotamine, other 5-HT agonists, lithium or some anti-depressants.

Naratriptan and sumatriptan should not be taken by anyone who has an allergy to sulphonamides. It is advisable to speak to your doctor or pharmacist about any other medication that you are taking whether it is on prescription or purchased over-the-counter.

Side-effects can include giddiness or pressure in the throat, chest or neck. Tingling of the limbs can be experienced as can a feeling of heaviness or weakness, increased sensitivity of the skin, dizziness or drowsiness and nausea. These side-effects, should they occur, should be mild and short-lasting.

Please remember that 5-HT agonists should not be taken daily to prevent attacks.

Prophylactic Drugs

Migraine prevention drugs have changed the lives of many sufferers. Patients who suffer frequent migraines, particularly if the attacks are severe and long lasting, need to consider the possibility of some form of prophylactic treatment.

Propranolol (brand name Inderal) is a commonly prescribed long term anti-migraine drug. It is a beta-blocker and as such belongs to a family of drugs which slow the heart rate and lower blood pressure. Although beta-blockers are used to treat high blood pressure, some have also been found to be useful in the treatment of migraine and propranolol is used especially for this condition. Another beta-blocker, atenolol (Tenormin), is often prescribed for use as a migraine preventative and works well for some sufferers. Asthmatics, patients with heart failure, people with severe chest problems and some diabetics are not recommended to take this drug. Side-effects include depression, nausea, insomnia and vivid dreams.

Pizotifen (brand name Sanomigran) was developed as a migraine preventative drug. It is a 5-HT blocker but it also has antihistamine properties. Side-effects include drowsiness and weight gain.

Another 5-HT blocker is methysergide (Deseril). Although it prevents attacks for many sufferers, it is not often prescribed these days because of its long list of possible side-effects which can include nausea, stomach pains, drowsiness, dizziness, restlessness, leg cramps, mood changes, vomiting, diarrhoea or constipation and ataxia (defective muscle control). Most important is the possibility of an irreversible side-effect following prolonged use of the drug; it may lead to fibrous thickening of the kidneys and other tissues. This has only been seen to happen in patients who take it continuously without the recommended one-month break for every six months of use. This is why it is usually prescribed under the supervision of a neurologist.

In spite of the many drawbacks, Deseril has helped many migraine sufferers. Patients who have previously had frequent very severe migraines are allowed to take Deseril for three to five months and then, to prevent the build up of unwanted side-effects, have to stop for a month before beginning the next course.

Calcium-Channel Blocker

This family of drugs is similar in action to the beta-blockers. They widen the blood vessels by relaxing the muscles in the vessel wall. Calcium-channel blockers are also used for the treatment of high blood pressure and some heart disease but unlike beta-blockers they can be used by asthma sufferers. Side-effects are mild and include drowsiness, weakness and weight gain. Nifedipine (brand name Adalat) is a calcium-channel blocker.

Clonidine

Marketed under the brand name of Dixarit this drug was first used in the treatment of high blood pressure. It is an alpha-agonist which affects the blood vessels, making them less sensitive to vasoactive amines and therefore less likely to dilate, says The Diamond Headache Clinic. Side-effects include drowsiness, constipation and depression.

Anti-depressants

Anti-depressants such as amitriptyline are often used in the prophylactic treatment of migraine, regardless of whether the patient is suffering from depression or not. There are different types of anti-depressants. One type of anti-depressant often prescribed for migraine sufferers is the tricyclics. These seem to work with patients even if depression is not a factor. Migraine sufferers have been found to have a high level of serotonin in their urine during attacks. Amitriptyline, brand name Tryptizol, is a mood elevator, working on the part of the brain that controls mood. But it also can make you drowsy and can cause dizziness and blurred vision. These symptoms are common in the early days of treatment, and the drug may not seem to be effective during this time. However, side-effects usually settle after a couple of weeks as the drug starts to take effect. It can also cause changes in the pulse, heart rhythm and blood pressure.

Anti-epilectics

The epilepsy drug sodium valproate (Epilim) is sometimes prescribed in low doses as a preventative for migraine. It does have side-effects but the main concern is that women must be using effective contraception because sodium valproate used in pregnancy is associated with a high rate of foetal abnormalities. That aside, it is worthwhile trying if migraine does not respond to other prophylactics.

Lithium

This light metal is sometimes used, in very small doses, for the treatment of chronic cluster headaches. For the treatment of mental illnesses like manic depression, it is used in much higher doses. It acts on nerve fibres by substituting for potassium, which occurs naturally in the body. Lithium takes several weeks before it starts to have an effect. Side-effects can include trembling, nausea, vomiting and diarrhoea.

12

The Psychological Angle

'Many patients consider their migraines to occur "spontaneously" and without cause. Such a view leads, scientifically, to absurdity, emotionally, to fatalism, and therapeutically, to impotence. We must assume that all attacks of migraine have real and discoverable determinants, however difficult their elucidation may be.' So says Dr Oliver Sacks in his book *Migraine*. Any doctor with that attitude is bound to be beloved of migraine patients. It is not so much the succeeding but the trying that is of the essence. And if this is what we want from our doctors, it is certainly what we should expect from ourselves. Putting up and shutting up is no way to cure an illness.

The trouble is that nowadays there are so many ways of tackling migraine that it is hard not to get confused. Practitioners of homoeopathy, acupuncture, reflexology, herbalism, allergy treatment and many others have helped migraine sufferers over the years, as have doctors practising traditional medicine. At the end of the day it doesn't matter where relief comes from as long as it has us out of the bedroom and back in the land of the living. So with that in mind, why don't we look at the most difficult, and sometimes the most painful, form of therapy – the one that has us looking closely into ourselves.

Repressed emotions

While researching this book I heard so many sufferers recall the bad times, when their migraine attacks were either very severe or very frequent. They would almost always add: 'I was under a lot of pressure at that time,' or 'It was an emotionally bad time.' This is borne out by study after study where migraine patients have said that emotional factors and stress figure very largely in triggering attacks. There are many theories that back up these findings, the most common of which is that a migraineur has inherited a predisposition to migraine. It is a weakness, if you like, which gets worse or reveals itself under physical or emotional stress.

But someone practising the 'talking' treatments like counselling, psychotherapy, behaviourism and so on would look at it from another perspective. They would examine the possibility that it was the behaviour pattern that had been inherited. If your mother, father or aunt reacted to stress or emotional upset by getting a migraine, the chances are that you may react to those conditions in the same way. And react means react – it doesn't mean 'putting it on'. It may be that in your family people didn't give full vent to their feelings. They didn't shout when they were angry, cry when they were unhappy and so on. It was an emotional control or bottling up that subconsciously found its release and expression in migraine, and over the generations it became a family tendency.

Here are two psychological aspects of migraine quoted from Dr Oliver Sacks's book *Migraine*:

Biologically the simplest, and dynamically the most benign of migraines, are recuperative. These tend to occur, circumstantially, following prolonged physical or emotional activity, and habitually as the notorious 'weekend' attacks. There is usually a rather sharp collapse from the preceding or provocative period of over-activity and tension, the phase of prostration may be profound and even stuporous, and it is followed, characteristically, by a post-migrainous rebound and sense of awakening re-animation.

Sounds familiar? How about this:

There are a number of patients in whom periodic or sporadic migraines are experienced which seem to embed, and to enact and 'work through' an accumulation of emotional stresses and conflicts. I have the impression that many menstrual migraines (and other allied menstrual syndromes) do exactly this, condensing, as it were, the stresses of the month into a few days of concentrated illness, and I have observed, in a number of patients, that curing them (depriving them) of such menstrual syndromes may be followed by a release of diffuse anxiety and conflict into the remainder of the month. Such migraines, in a word, may serve to bind, and thus circumscribe, painful, chronic or recurrent feelings, a consideration which must be borne in mind before they are too zealously dispersed.

Do some of us get migraines because it is the only way in which we can express our hurt, anger and frustrations? Do some of us get them because it is the only way in which we can allow ourselves to get away from it all and rest? These questions may sound far-fetched, or they may ring a faint bell; either way, it's worth keeping an open mind about the cause of migraine. It could be body chemistry. It could be the result of something buried in the psyche. It's very possibly a combination.

So how do you tackle the psychological part? A trained therapist or counsellor can help you look inwards and discover how you handle emotional situations and relationships. Let's just take an example: do you give as good as you get, or are you constantly on the receiving end of other people's anger and frustrations? Do you shrug it off in an attempt to convince yourself that it doesn't matter anyway – when it does? And as a result does it fester away in your subconscious? If this strikes a chord, you can be sure you are one of a very large crowd. Expert help can enable you to see what is happening and give you the confidence to act in a way that's best for you – not for the other person. That could mean handing back the anger to the owner and making sure that you are not saddled with it. That kind of liberation can take the punch out of your migraines, even if it does not cure them.

Childhood legacies

A psychoanalyst or therapist may want to draw back the curtains further and look more deeply into your childhood. After all, there is a reason why we behave the way we do, and it very often dates back to something that happened when we were children. Why don't you have the confidence to shout back, tell people to get lost or refuse to do things that you don't want to do? Maybe you are naturally submissive. Maybe you were brought up to be seen and not heard. Maybe it is the result of some unresolved fear buried deep in your psyche. Fear in childhood is not uncommon, but if it becomes traumatic and unresolved it can haunt our adult lives – and people often do not know that it is even there. This kind of deep digging can be difficult, time-consuming and costly, but the therapy exists and it does work for some people.

Depression

Many headaches are accompanied by chronic depression and migraine and depression are often seen together. Some of the early signs of depression are sleep disturbance, along with a loss of concentration, appetite or interest in anything. A depressed person may also suffer constant fatigue and stomach pains. He or she will be irritable and tearful. Untreated, depression and migraine can become a vicious circle. You suffer from depression because you get migraines, and you get migraines because you are depressed. Antidepressants are often used in the prophylactic treatment of migraines, even for patients who are not depressed. The theory, according to the Diamond Headache Clinic, is that any form of treatment that has a beneficial effect on the emotions should also lessen the frequency of migraine attacks. However, patients suffering from depression would do well to consider one of the talking treatments. Baring your soul to a counsellor trained to listen could effectively break the circle.

Curiously, migraine sufferers (and sufferers from other chronic illnesses) very often don't get attacks if they are in extremely stressful conditions or severe clinical depression. In Chapter 1, Cynthia commented that while she was 'in the pit' she didn't have a single migraine; they only came back when she started to climb out.

In his book *Migraine*, Dr Oliver Sacks relates the case history of a man who had suffered from migraines since the age of seven until he was imprisoned in Auschwitz during World War Two. Throughout his six years in the concentration camp, during which time his wife and parents and all his close relatives were killed, he did not suffer a single migraine. In the decades since his liberation he has suffered from chronic depression along with feelings of guilt; he gets on average six-to-ten severe attacks of classical migraine every month. He is apparently accident-prone, and his only respites from migraine are when he has injured himself badly or when his depression is so acute that he has to go into hospital for treatment.

Elizabeth suffered from weekend migraines, and would spend most Saturday and Sundays 'feeling grim'. She would get a throbbing headache, sometimes accompanied by sickness. None of the drugs she was offered had much effect. During this time she was having a problematical relationship with a man – for ten years or more they could not make up their minds whether to get married. The trouble was, says Elizabeth, that they found it difficult to talk about anything personal. She started having counselling, and she says: 'I had this image of exploding dustbins. You stuff all this down into the dustbins and then you sit on the lid and now and again it explodes.' A year ago she started seeing a psychotherapist.

Elizabeth

She asked me why I had come to see her. I said that I wanted to get rid of my migraines. And she said: 'Oh, I can help you do that.' She was the first person who had said that to me. 'Oh yes,' she said. 'I used to have a lot of migraines. I don't get any now.'

I saw her once a week for an hour each time. We spent a lot of time talking about childhood and talking about the relationship – what had gone wrong with it. The sexual side, which I hadn't really gone into or thought about or acknowledged. I was having menstrual problems and I came off the Pill, and that was the end of the sexual side of our relationship because he wasn't prepared to do anything about it. And we weren't able to talk about it. That lasted for three years. I can't imagine it really now. In my mind it started to fit together. Looking back he'd come round on a Friday and on the Saturday I'd get a migraine.

One of the problems that was carried over from childhood was my wariness of getting close to people – of really telling them what was bugging me. My father's attitude was: 'If you don't stop crying I'll give you something to cry for.' I still hear that voice. My mother died this summer, and I was aware that I didn't want to get close to her and she certainly didn't get close to me. So I think from childhood there was that pattern of bottling it all up inside.

I think the psychotherapy has been a way of saying it is all right to talk about these things. Being able to talk through both childhood experiences and problems with relationships. I think the two have gone together. The problems in the relationship were determined partly by problems that were carried over from childhood.

I saw it then as his unwillingness to talk about things, but it was probably my unwillingness as well. We didn't really want to talk about what the root of the problem was.

I was also a workaholic, which perhaps contributed to the problems in the relationship. Everything had to be 'just so'. I worked every evening until about ten o'clock and I worked all Saturday and most of Sunday.

There was a time when the relationship was ending when I just went to pieces. I sat around at home for a week crying. I couldn't understand what was going on, but I think it was my whole body saying: 'This is enough. Work is enough. The relationship is enough.' I'd always been a churchgoer but God seemed to have disappeared off the scene. There was nothing left. I spent about six months of that year being really depressed. That was when I first had counselling from one of the ministers of my church. He really bailed me out because I was quite suicidal at times.

A couple of weeks before she died, my mother went into a home. I was just about to take her out in the wheelchair to look at the sea when she said, quite out of the blue: 'I've only just realized how much Dad loved me. And I was always so cold towards him.' I nearly fell through the floor. I thought how sad. It counts for so much. They didn't have a very positive sexual relationship. He was a very fiery-tempered man. I never took friends home as a child in case he was in a bad mood. My mother never had friends round to tea just in case he came back from work.

My mother was quite protective towards me. She would fend off father. She was protective, but not close. I never confided in her.

Taking the lid off things has actually helped. I had an argument with somebody yesterday. I was really fuming and I thought: 'This is exactly the situation where tomorrow I'll have a migraine.' And then I thought:

I'll go and talk to somebody.' So I exploded over a couple of people I came across. I couldn't have done that years ago. I would have just kept it all bottled up.

I think the turning point came for me one day when the psychotherapist asked: 'How do you feel now?' and I said: 'I don't know. I feel like a balloon that's tied down with lots and lots of string.'

She said: 'What colour is it? and I said. 'It's red.'

Her parting shot was: 'Why don't you go home and write the story of the red balloon?' I got some nice paper and I folded it to make a little book and I just sat and wrote it. I didn't know what I was going to write. It was just the story of the red balloon. Then I read it and I just sat there and cried. It was terribly important.

I started writing lots of poems and painting pictures and things after that. And it's been a tremendous help in terms of exploring the inner world. I found things have come out that I didn't know were inside. They are there to be talked about. It helps to heal memories. As long as I can't talk about it, it remains there as an exploding dustbin. Then you talk about something with great difficulty and next week you think: 'Why was that so difficult to talk about?' And you end up having a good laugh about it.

Elizabeth's migraines are very few and far between these days. She has given up her career at which she was very successful but worked extremely hard, and she is now a full-time student embarking on a very different type of professional life. Although the relationship has ended, she is still in touch with her friend.

Richard is a highly skilled and very experienced analytical psychologist. He also suffered from severe classical migraine attacks, which he cured through analysis: he was able to look behind the zigzags and flashing lights and see the ghost of his childhood hiding there.

Richard
Although I didn't realize it, I think I was having migraine attacks from very early on as a child in South Africa. Certainly I was having incapacitating bilious attacks. I can remember only wanting to be in a darkened room, and a very powerful feeling of pressure and anxiety. It wasn't really until my university days that I became aware of it in the standard or classical form.

It would start with a spot – a dot literally somewhere in the visual field. I would tend to want to focus away from it altogether. That would gradually spread into a kaleidoscope of black and white flashing rings which expanded slowly. But prior to that, almost before it happened, I'd become aware of problems with my vision. There would be areas out of sync. I'd feel as if I was seeing half a person or half a face. And it would come and go. The thing would expand until it covered the whole of my vision. I wouldn't be totally blind – I could see through it and around it.

The visual symptoms were positively terrifying. One was losing some sort of controlling contact with the world, really. I found there was a strange kind of alteration in the way things sounded – an echo chamber sort of thing. In some ways one felt it was a kind of doubling going on – visually as well as orally. It's a fearful experience to have your vision interfered with. It's not just a straightforward 'I'm going blind' type of thing. Fear is very much part of it.

When I knew more about psychology I experimented with it. I wanted to see how much one could work with it and see with it. I played tennis while I had the aura; and I got people to throw things at me and I caught them. It was very interesting, because basically the aura didn't seem to alter my co-ordination. It wasn't at all pleasant to do, but I could catch the ball. I couldn't actually see it. It would just vanish, but I'd catch it. The stress was pretty heavy at these times, because I was battling against a very powerful desire to get into the dark and shut off all stimuli.

The aura would last about twenty minutes. Then there would be a break when I'd still feel lousy, and then the headache would start. Sometimes there was quite a clear period in between in which everything was very clear – almost as if one had come out into a clarity one didn't have before. It nearly always led to tremendous nausea, vomiting and so on which lasted for most of the day. By the next morning it would be OK, but I'd be feeling pretty precarious. Even as a child the bilious attacks would incapacitate me. My mother's reaction to it was castor oil, I think.

My real time of migraine attacks was after the war when I was doing three things at once. I was doing a private practice as a psychologist and I was running a clinic and I was lecturing. When that got really heavy my migraines were at their worst. I tried everything I could think of. I became aware then of what I could only describe as hypoglycaemic attacks – really severe feelings of sudden loss of blood sugar, I suppose. Coldness inside, a feeling of impending death. Terrifying feelings. I started taking glucose and things of this kind to see if they would help. They didn't. It became very severe. I had one attack which developed almost into the shakes, coupled with exhaustion. From that point on they put me on very small doses of phenobarbitone. It didn't do anything for me, as far as I can remember, apart from make me feel that I was looking at everything through a curtain.

Then I started going to an analyst in Durban. It was part of the training. It didn't help me greatly. I think it was my fault. I am sure I controlled that thoroughly. I didn't allow the analysis to get to me. I produced the right dreams and I did the right things, but I'm not sure that I changed very much underneath at all.

I got a fellowship which enabled me to come to London with the family and I was able to do the final two years of my training in England. As part of my training I saw an analyst who was really quite something. She tied me up in knots straightaway, and there was no way in which I could keep my defences with her. She really broke through. It was during that two and a half years that the migraines literally disappeared. I went through certain very strange experiences with her.

It was as if I was suddenly in that very clear thing – like the period after the aura and before the headache. Only it was without any aura and without any headache. It hit me for about a week. I suddenly found myself seeing everything differently. Everything was astonishingly clear. Frighteningly clear. The scenery, the people – it was very visual. If I had been having LSD or something like that I could have understood it a bit better, but it was as if everything was brighter, more shiny, clearer, precise and so on. It didn't feel right. It felt very weird. I went along to my analyst about this and her only response was 'a psychotic episode wouldn't do you any harm'. She was right, of course.

It was very important for me to get down behind whatever these cautious controls of mine were. I started to feel that what was going on in the aura was not just an interference with my vision – it was as if there was something else trying to impose itself on my vision other than what I was looking at. I myself was producing some of the kaleidoscopic effect to obscure this. When this was happening I tried quite seriously to see behind it. I did get various impressions. I can't say I actually saw things. But I had various impressions about very early experiences of separation from my mother particularly. I had been separated early on, going to my grandfather's farm. She would come out, leave me there and go back to my father, because he never came to the farm. This was during all the holiday times, sometimes for weeks or months. I became aware of those times and of very deep feelings of deprivation and darkness when I was trying to look through this thing.

One of the reasons I did this was because my analyst had done some extraordinary work with epileptics and she'd been able to get them to express their attacks in psychological terms. She got them to draw and to paint when they got an aura. She had enabled them to find ways in which they could translate whatever this sparking was that was going on inside into forms which they could put on to paper. She had enabled a number of them to reduce or prevent their attacks.

When I was having an attack I tried literally to see if there was another picture that the flashes and kaleidoscopic effect were really trying to block out. One image I got was of myself as a very weedy little creature floating around unattached to anything, thoroughly pathetic. It was definitely very much the abandoned child sort of emotion which was in it. There was absolute terror, total disconnection and maybe there was rage in it too. It is very difficult ever to say that that was the cause of the migraines. But certainly as I went through my analysis the migraines did reduce, and finally they disappeared with very few exceptions.

At the end of the two-and-a-half years I couldn't stay on. I had to go back to South Africa. I think I may have had two or three attacks of migraine over the next two or three years.

In South Africa we went through an awful lot of strain because of apartheid. I was running a multi-racial clinic. We were under threat all the time. The tension was very high. We were regularly visited by the security police, who took all our files on one occasion and so on. So we stopped taking notes. From the time I went back it was a question of do I stay on or not. We were seeing in the one clinic Africans, Asians, blacks and whites, which was very much against the rules. They should all have been in separate clinics. Eventually that was forced on us and that's when I left. However, during this time my migraines didn't build up again although I was working very hard. I had to save money because I felt that the chances were I would have to go. I wasn't sure what money I would be able to take with me. I was in a fortunate position because I was also a British citizen.

In 1962 I came back here. The old tensions were gone and I felt an oasis of calm. I had the problems of establishing myself, but there was no rush about anything. I didn't get migraines although it was tricky settling down.

I feel I looked at what the migraine was about and got rid of some of the predisposition to it. I felt my analysis did do a lot for it. Since I left South Africa I have had a lot of depressed feelings and things of that sort. I think it's about leaving things over there and being dispossessed to some extent. I think for me it was the abandonment feeling – this loss of mother and terror engendered by that. In a way I can still feel some of that terror now, but possibly the fact that I can feel it is why I don't get migraine.

Bridget suffered from acidosis as a child – a condition in which greater than normal amounts of acid appear in the blood. This gave way in later years to migraine. Bridget puts the condition down to stress. When you read the story of her childhood you will understand why.

Bridget

With the help of the Migraine Action Association I did work out, during the migraine years, most of the trigger factors affecting me and I did work my way through a lot of unhelpful drugs until I found ergotamine. Now, the migraine trigger factors are very complicated and usually multiple, but one very constant factor is that I have to have been under recent, severe stress.

Going back to the acidosis years, I should say that ninety per cent of that was stress-related. I had an elder brother and was the least important member of a violent and hysterical family. My father had a very violent temper which often led to kicks and blows, and more often still to imminent fear of kicks and blows. But you know how it is – you remember odd incidents from childhood and it's difficult to say exactly how often he hit me. My mother also hit me, but more often she would threaten me with a stick or get my father to hit me. I can only say that as early as I can remember I learned to stay out of the way of the rest of my family, hiding in cupboards, behind my bed, up trees etc. I used to take books with me to these places. In fact I'm sure that's why I learned enough to pass my exams.

My mother never tried to protect me from my father's violence. On the contrary, she was a manipulative schemer who devoted, so I can see now, considerable effort to making trouble between my father and me. She certainly never tried to stop him or to console me. Furthermore she encouraged my older brother to join in the fun, and I can remember to this day the regular hard punches he would give me in the stomach, completely winding me.

When I was about five and my brother eight I was accused of trying to murder him. We were in the back of our old car and my parents in the front. I had, as usual, been lost in my own thoughts when I suddenly noticed, and immediately cried out to my parents, that my brother was no longer sitting on his side of the seat but was lying curled up on the floor on his side with his head apparently under my father's seat. My father slammed the brakes on and leaped out of the car. I remember another car hooting at him for stopping so suddenly and for opening the door without looking. I don't recall that there was anything wrong with my brother other than that he was whimpering a bit. It was my father who accused me of trying to kill him by pushing him down under the seat and throwing a blanket down on top of him. It was, of course, a ridiculous accusation as he was older, bigger and much rougher than I was and he had not cried out in protest at any stage. No one challenged it however and it passed into family mythology.

The atmosphere at mealtimes was unendurable. My mother's very rich food – she had been a professional cook before she married – left me bent over with acidosis after about two mouthfuls. I actually found it very difficult to swallow anything except tea and raw fruit. She was keen on cream, butter, meat, eggs and fat, with everything beaten and sieved as smooth as possible. Inevitably both my parents died of strokes. I was, of course, very thin. If my father was violent he would try to kick me under the table and I used to have to sit with my legs folded up as high as I could hold them to keep them out of the way. To this day I do not like eating in company – even with my own husband and daughter.

When I got to Oxford – all that reading did me good – to my surprise I found I could eat without getting colic. I put this down to the change of diet from rich to plain, but looking back on it I think it probably had more to do with the relative lack of stress. I did get migraines and I did also have often to stop eating after a mouthful or two because my stomach suddenly tied itself into a knot, but on the whole I had a great time. However, I never did catch the trick of eating sensibly. As the years passed I found I could actually eat a whole meal and enjoy it and not get colic, nor, most of the time, a migraine. I think I may subconsciously have tried to make up for lost time. I began to snack instead of eating proper meals. I ate all the sweet and starchy things I had never been able to manage before and I began to put on weight.

I am a tall person and I started adulthood very thin indeed, so it took years to become seriously fat, but I am now very overweight and mildly diabetic. I simply cannot persuade myself to eat properly.

That is as far as I have got. I am not currently under stress, or to be more exact there is no current factor causing stress. But I find I can't, as I had hoped, simply put my family behind me and forget them. My parents are dead and I take good care never to see my brother. But I can't stop myself thinking about them and how awful they were, and just the thoughts make me very stressed.

Both Herta's mother and grandmother suffered from migraines. Herta's own migraines started when she was forty-five. She was told that they would get better as she got older, but at sixty-five she's still waiting. She has migraines without aura but with dizziness, nausea, light sensitivity and the rest of it. She has been down the food allergy road, giving up yeast and milk products, carrots, green beans, sweet-corn and anything she thought might be provocative, with 'the intense will to make it better'. At one time she was experiencing an attack every week and each attack lasted three days. Now, with the help of Sanomigran, things are better.

Herta does not feel that her migraines are connected to her child-hood. After all, they took forty-five years to come. But the latter part of her childhood was extraordinary, to say the least, and in some ways reminiscent of the feelings of fear and abandonment that Richard talked about earlier.

Herta is a Viennese Jewess. Before the start of World War Two, she and her brother came over to England with the Children's Transports, a scheme by which some Jewish children were brought out of Austria and placed with British families. She was twelve years old at the time.

Herta

My parents could not get permission to come out, so they were left in Vienna. Mother was highly pregnant with my youngest brother who was born over there.

I can remember my nightmare. Jews were not going to be picked up by the ambulance. I was afraid that my mother would have the baby and be bleeding to death in the road. In fact the birth was all right.

A family in Liverpool said that they would take both myself and my brother in. We went to school – not understanding a word. The war started and we were evacuated to Chester with a different family. One family took my brother and one family took me. My brother's nightmare was waking up in the middle of the night knowing that Mother and Father were roaming the streets, not knowing where their children were, and they said to themselves: 'The next light that goes on will be where they live.' So he got up and switched the light on.

My parents got out in August 1939 and they came over as domestics. They lived in poky lodgings with a six-month-old baby. Eventually my little brother was put into a home. They used to visit him once a week. When I got to the age of fourteen in Chester I took myself off to London to live with my parents again, not realizing that they lived in a small bedsit and didn't have room for another bed. The landlady very kindly let them have another poky little room upstairs where I slept. To me it was heaven. I went out to work in the clothing trade as a cutter's assistant. I stood for nine hours a day at the cutting table except for tea and lunch breaks. They were on a wartime contract.

I'm a positive thinker – I'd rather think of the positive things that come out of tragedy. I met my husband in a youth club in London called Young Austria. He didn't know what had happened to his parents. We got married when I was eighteen and he was twenty-one. Later we were able to trace through archives in Israel what had happened to my husband's parents. We found the date of the transport. They never actually got into the camp at Auschwitz. They went straight to the gas chamber. So we know when it happened. It was in October and we were married that November. Of course at the time we had no idea at all. But there is continuity. And I believe greatly in that.

13

Alternative Therapies

There are a number of treatments available in Britain which do not rely on drugs or surgery. Many of the alternative therapies claim to treat the person – not the disease. In Chinese medicine, for instance the doctor will look at the way you walk into the room, your posture, complexion and so on to get a picture of you as a person. As with other forms of treatment, it is very important to go to a qualified practitioner. However, there are no laws governing complementary medicine in Britain at present, so anyone can set themselves up. This situation would create a minefield except for the fact that therapists tend to belong to the appropriate professional body, which usually requires its members to have pass examinations and reached the required standard. So unless you are personally recommended to see a particular doctor or therapist don't pick one at random. Contact the relevant professional body and ask them to recommend one in your area. Remember that most complementary medicine is not available on the National Health, so it is well worth finding out the likely cost before embarking on any treatment.

This chapter describes some of the therapies that claim to be able to help migraine patients. Names and addresses of professional bodies are listed in the Useful Addresses section.

Since so much of complementary medicine is outside scientific definition and proof, how you feel about any particular therapy is important – more so than with traditional medicine. However many of these therapies say that the patient does not have to believe that it is going to work for it to do so. But it does help to have some respect for the treatment involved and to relate to it in a positive way.

There is no 'right' treatment, but there is almost certainly a right treatment for you. This might be traditional medicine, counselling psychotherapy or one of the many complementary treatments and medicines on offer. I have therefore made no attempt to compare these alternative treatments or to analyse or criticize them. So read the descriptions given here and see if anything appeals to you. There are many dimensions to migraine – in the way we each experience the illness and also in the way each one of us goes about treating it.

Two of the treatments described here, chiropractic and osteopathy, have been successfully tried by members of the Migraine

Action Association and their stories appear along with the therapy. The herbal remedy feverfew also appears in this section, along with a member's story.

Acupuncture

The English word 'acupuncture' means literally 'needle piercing'. In China, where this treatment is practised widely, it is called Chen chiu, which means 'needle moxa'. Moxa is a dried herb which is burned in small cones on the skin or on the handle of the needle to generate a gentle heat. This method is known as moxibustion. Both these methods can be used during the course of acupuncture treatment.

Since the needles are so fine there is no discomfort during the treatment, but patients may feel a slight tingling. The needles may be left in for twenty minutes to half an hour, or they may be withdrawn immediately. The moxa is burned on, or held near to the point, and removed when the patient feels that it is becoming too hot. This process is repeated several times.

Children or adults who have a fear of needles are usually given another form of treatment. This includes massage and tapping or pressure with a rounded probe. Alternatively they may receive electro-acupuncture and laser treatments in which the acupuncture points are stimulated either by a low frequency electrical current, applied direct with a probe, or with finely tuned laser beams. Gentle electrical stimuli may also be applied through the needles, giving a sensation of tingling or buzzing.

Acupuncture is part of a system of medicine that has been practised in China for several thousand years. More recently its use has been popularized worldwide and research has taken place into the whys and wherefores of its efficacy. One discovery has been that stimulation of acupuncture points induces the release by the brain of pain-relieving morphine-like substances known as endorphins. This may explain why acupuncture has been used so successfully as an alternative to anaesthetics in surgery.

Acupuncture is based on the principle that our health depends on the balanced functioning of the body's motivating energy known as Chi, this energy flows throughout the body but is concentrated in channels beneath the skin. These channels are called meridians and along them lie the points by which the acupuncturist regulates the energy flow and bodily health.

The treatment aims to restore the harmony between the equal and opposite qualities of chi, the *yang* and the *yin*. Yang energy is aggressive, representing light, heat, dryness and contraction. Yin energy is receptive, representing tranquillity, darkness, coldness moisture and swelling. A dominance of yang energy in the body is thought to be experienced in the form of acute pain, headache, inflammation, spasms and high blood pressure. An excess of yin felt as dull aches and pains, chilliness, fluid retention, discharges and fatigue.

Practitioners of acupuncture aim to discover the nature of the disharmony in the body. They do this by careful questioning and observation: they will examine the patient's tongue for its structure, colour and coating, and feel the pulses for their quality and strength. Once the cause of the problem has been diagnosed, the acupuncturist will select the points and the appropriate method of treatment. Apart from its pain-relieving and relaxing effects, acupuncture aims to restore the balance of the energy system, thus enabling the body's self-healing mechanism to work better.

Some GPs practise acupuncture in their surgeries. Others will be able to recommend a qualified practitioner. If you don't want to go through your GP, you can find a qualified practitioner through the professional societies. Since needles are involved in the treatment, the big question mark is going to be hepatitis and AIDS. Members of these professional bodies have to use needle sterilization techniques approved by the Department of Health. These are considered to be effective against the hepatitis and AIDS viruses. Many practitioners use disposable needles.

The Alexander technique

Patients with tension headaches and migraines which affect the neck and shoulders may be interested in this method of self-help which involves teaching your body how to obviate such problems. The Alexander technique is a way of unlearning bad habits in sitting, standing, walking – in fact any way you move or stay still – and replacing them with a better way of using your body. This in turn helps relieve tension pains in the back, neck, shoulders and many other places in the body.

The idea is that when the body is working the way it should there is less drag and inefficiency, and as the various parts of the body gain greater freedom improvements are felt in breathing, circulation and digestion. Teachers of the technique say that as people learn to use their bodies in a more natural way many problems brought about by stress can be resolved. If the way you sit, stand, walk or sleep creates unnecessary muscular stress and tension, this will adversely affect your general well-being. Stressing the neck and shoulder muscles is likely to have a knock-on effect on muscles in the face and head. Since migraine is, for some sufferers, so stress – and tension-related, this technique is worth considering.

It was evolved by an Australian actor called Frederick Matthias Alexander, who found that when he gave a performance his voice would very quickly become hoarse. Since no medical help worked for him, he began to study the way in which he misused his vocal mechanisms and his body as a whole. Gradually he taught himself to prevent this misuse and overcame this embarrassing disability.

After further study he came to realize that all our activities are dependent for their efficiency on a proper relationship of the head, neck and back. If this is achieved, a muscular harmony throughout the body follows. If it isn't the whole system becomes disorganized.

The head should lead the body, and not the other way around. The head should be balanced on top of the spinal column by the appropriate small muscles, and not held by the larger outside muscles of the neck. When these large muscles usurp the function of the smaller ones, shortening and narrowing of the back occurs and muscular imbalance takes place throughout the body.

So the technique lies not so much in teaching you how to sit or stand properly as in teaching you how to use your body in a natural and beneficial way. Apparently most of us lose this ability as little children by copying the bad habits of our elders! This is then aggravated through the pressures of daily living.

The aim is to teach people how to get their own natural, inborn postural reflexes going again. The teacher gently guides the body into the most natural state – there is no spinal manipulation or physical discomfort. The idea is to help the student to find the necessary degree of muscle tension required to support the body against the downward pull of gravity. One of the by-products of mastering the technique is that you are able to stand and walk tall without stiffness.

Part of the course consists of verbal instruction. The student is taught to become conscious of the way in which he is misusing his body, and learns to project simple messages from the brain to the body to help prevent it.

To learn all this is not easy, and you will not master the technique overnight. Lessons last between thirty-to-forty minutes and you may need twenty-to-thirty lessons spread over three-to-five months.

Aromatherapy

Practised widely in France, aromatherapy has been gaining a name for itself in Britain for the treatment of stress-related illnesses, including migraine. Instead of drugs this therapy uses essential plant oils. An essential oil is what gives fragrance to a flower or herb. It is a liquid which is present in tiny droplets in the plants. Each essential oil has a number of different properties, and it is the aromatherapist's job to evaluate which oil or mixture of oils will have a beneficial effect on a particular condition. For instance some of the essential oils can have powerful antibiotic properties, while others are effective with psychotherapeutic conditions such as insomnia, migraine and headaches, depression and pre-menstrual syndrome.

The essential oils are used in a variety of different ways. They can be massaged into the body, or used in compresses, inhalations and vaporizers or even in the bath.

With migraine there is the problem of smell. If smell is a trigger, should you give this therapy a miss? Aromatherapists say that migraine responds well to this treatment, but if smell affects you it is best not to have the first treatment when you know an attack is impending.

A trained aromatherapist will try and work out with you, if possible, the underlying cause of the migraines. If, for instance, they are menstrually related, the therapist will find an oil or a combination of oils to treat the menstrual condition. Lovage is apparently a very good oil for menstrual migraines. If the basis of the migraines is digestive, the therapist will aim to sort that out and in so doing alleviate the migraine. Stress-related migraines respond well to lavender oil. In fact some sufferers say that a sniff of lavender at the start of an attack can abort it within ten minutes. However, it is unlikely to work for everybody. People do have an affinity to a certain smell or smells, say the aromatherapists, and that would be the right essential oil or blend for them.

Although you can use aromatherapy on yourself there are definite advantages in seeing an aromatherapist, particularly for an important condition like migraine. Apart from the fact that he or she should be trained to mix a cocktail of oils that is specifically beneficial to you, they can give you something you cannot do yourself – a good massage. Massage has many benefits. It stimulates the circulation of blood and lymph. It can reduce high blood pressure, stimulate the immune system and reduce muscular tension. Massage can also reduce swelling and pain in muscles and joints – many aromatherapy patients find this the best part of the treatment because it soothes and revitalizes them.

Of course seeing a therapist is much more expensive than do-it-yourself treatment, and aromatherapy needs to be maintained at home. Probably the best bet would be to go to a qualified aroma-therapist for a thorough consultation. You will then be given the oils you need in cream, lotion and/or inhalation form to use at home. You can then have a massage as, when and if the wallet is willing!

Chiropractic

The word 'chiropractic' originates from the Greek words *cheiro*, hand, and *praktos*, to use; so it means 'done by hand'. As far as migraines are concerned, it is thought that stiff spinal joints can create tension in the neck muscles which in turn can cause headaches and migraine.

Chiropractors believe that the body is a machine, with the spine its most important part. If the spine gets damaged, distorted or irritated, trouble starts. Even a minor displacement of the spine can cause problems. Over a period of five years chiropractors are trained to look for spinal nerve stress or vertebral displacements, which they do with the help of X-rays. After identifying spinal nerve stress, the chiropractor uses specific chiropractic adjustment to correct the condition and relieve the stress. When this is achieved, the body is able to restore itself to normality. This freeing of spinal stress, chiropractors believe, particularly in the cervical spine or neck, can bring lasting relief to headache sufferers.

Ten-year-old Corinne, whose story appears below, was cured of her migraines through chiropractic. If you would like to know more about this therapy and find a chiropractor, your GP may well be able to help as can the British Chiropractic Association.

Corinne
(as told by her mother)
After a bit of flu in November my ten-year-old developed sinusitis, which didn't seem to respond to six different antibiotics. She then started to have severe migraines, several each week, some of which were bad enough to temporarily paralyse her. After X-rays the doctors told us the sinuses were not badly blocked and nothing should be done – it would all go away eventually. She would grow out of it.

By mid-February we were desperate. We paid privately to see a neurologist, who gave her a brain scan and some propranolol tablets. He said virtually the same as the other doctors. Once the sinuses had sorted themselves out she would be all right. Corinne had been off school all this time. The worry of being off school probably contributed to the frequency of the migraines. The tablets had no effect. In desperation I took her to a chiropractor I was recommended to see by a friend.

She seemed to think that all sorts of things weren't right in her neck and her back, and this was probably related to a fall that she'd had just before the flu. At the time she had complained of a stiff neck and stiff shoulders. It then seemed to go and we didn't think any more of it.

The doctors had all twisted her neck and felt down her neck superficially. With the chiropractor the examination took a long time. She reorganized Corinne's back and neck and did what I believe she called 'cranial manipulation'. The first time she adjusted the neck we noticed an improvement. Corinne said she felt very much better. It ready seemed to perk her up. But going back in the car we had to stop. Corinne thought she was going to be sick. She started coughing up enormous amounts of sinus fluid. Every time we went back for treatment this happened, but the treatment itself was gentle.

The chiropractor said that because her neck had been out for so long it might not stay where it should be. So we went back weekly. Corinne still had the headaches, but immediately after going to the chiropractor and releasing some of this stuff she seemed to be that much better. However it only seemed to be temporary relief. The chiropractor noticed that Corinne had a tooth growing at right angles to the others, protruding almost into the roof of her mouth. She told us that if we had this out her neck would stay as it should be and she would make better progress.

Corinne had the tooth removed, although the dentist didn't believe it was causing any problems. She had the most almighty migraine that night. She was so ill she screamed for a long time. I thought that that was peculiar, because whenever I've had a migraine I've always wanted to keep absolutely quiet and silent and not move. But she just screamed. We had my mother-in-law staying here as well because I was finding it such a strain. She said she'd never seen anything like it. It was three-quarters of an hour before it subsided, and then she slept.

I was afraid that taking the tooth out might have made things worse, but within a couple of weeks she was completely cured. Every last trace of the sinus problem cleared and the migraines ceased. The chiropractor told us that the tooth appeared to be buckling the roof of the mouth, which is in effect the base of the skull, and it was throwing everything out of alignment.

So Corinne's migraines were a combination of several things, and however long we had waited I don't think they would have gone away on their own. The chiropractor told us of several cases of people suffering from headaches of one form or another which had been completely cured by realigning what appears to be some totally different part of the body. It appears that some seemingly minor injuries like my daughter's can cause all sorts of problems.

I hope that our story is of use to someone. I think the message is 'Don't ever give up hope' and try anything within reason.

Feverfew

The perennial plant feverfew (*Tanacetum parthenium*) grows wild in Europe but can also be cultivated. It grows to a height of between 14 and 45cm, and has strong-smelling greenish yellow leaves which taste bitter. The daisy-like flowers have white outer petals and yellow centres. There is also a double variety.

To prevent migraine one large or three smaller leaves are eaten daily. This amount can be chopped and eaten in a sandwich – some people sprinkle sugar on to take away the bitter taste. A small leaf is one measuring about 3cm by 3cm.

A trial of wild feverfew carried out at the City of London Migraine Clinic found that it reduced the frequency and/or severity of migraine attacks in approximately 70 per cent of users. Patients who had taken part in this trial had been on feverfew for some time and tolerated it well. However, a survey of three hundred users of the herb found that 18 per cent reported adverse side-effects, the most troublesome of which was mouth ulcers (11 per cent). Feverfew in any form can cause inflammation of the mouth and tongue and swelling of the lips.

Whether or not it is safe to take feverfew for long periods is not fully known. Pregnant women should avoid it, since it has not yet been established whether the plant has any effect on the unborn child. In the old days this herb was used to help expel a stillborn child, and it is also said to cause cattle to abort. No research has been done into the effects of feverfew on young children, so it should not be given to anyone under the age of twelve. The herb should also be avoided by nursing mothers.

Various brands of feverfew tablets and capsules are sold in chemists and health shops. Some of these contain quite large amounts of the dried herb. One small leaf is approximately 25mg when dried, so you can work out a suitable dose, bearing in mind that the smallest effective dose is the safest.

If you want to grow your own, you can get the seeds from reputable seed merchants. However, if someone offers you feverfew plants from their garden make sure that they really are feverfew. To ensure a good supply of leaves, three or more plants should be grown. Feverfew can be grown in any soil and does best in semi-shade. One of the three plants should be allowed to flower in order to get seeds for new plants. The other two should be kept for their daily supply of leaves. In order to keep up the strength and number of leaves, remove the flower heads of these two plants so that they do not develop seeds. Since it is a perennial, feverfew is also available during the winter. A little protection may be necessary in very cold weather. It can be potted and brought indoors if necessary. Leaves for taking on holiday can be picked beforehand and kept in water, but they will not keep for long.

However, dried feverfew seems to work as well as the fresh leaves. To get the best results pick the leaves on a dry sunny day, after the dew has dried. As soon as you have picked them, spread them out in a single layer in a well-ventilated place, out of direct sunlight. For the first few days keep turning them over so that they dry evenly and thoroughly. When they are completely dry, store the leaves, still whole if possible, in a tin or glass jar with a lid.

Dried feverfew can be eaten in the same way as the fresh leaves, but it is not recommended to be taken in an infusion or 'tea' as the amount and strength of each dose can be difficult to control when it is taken in this way. It is possible to buy 'chrysanthemum tea' which is sometimes called 'dried' feverfew, but as this is often imported and cannot be guaranteed to be pure feverfew, it is probably best to give it a miss.

April has suffered from migraines since she was sixteen. She had them throughout her pregnancies, and a subsequent hysterectomy has made no difference. She gets mini-attacks about twice a week but she can carry on through them. However, the major attacks, which come every two months, last for three days during which time she can be very sick. Anti-sickness tablets didn't help, and Cafergot suppositories worked sometimes but not always. She tends to rely on Migraleve, and nowadays feverfew.

April

One of the worst attacks I've had was on my daughter's wedding day. It was a traumatic time in our lives. My husband had been made redundant and he'd tried a series of jobs that hadn't worked out. We decided to move and we bought a business. The day we moved I knew that we were doing the wrong thing.

My daughter's wedding day came and the night before I put a party on. I didn't over-drink, because you can't with migraine. You know darn well that if you have more than a couple of glasses you're going to get a migraine. The next morning came and I couldn't believe it, I felt absolutely dreadful. I was being sick. At half-past-one I was in bed being sick, and at half-past-two she was getting married.

I had these Cafergot suppositories and I'd used about three of those by that time. My husband got me dressed. I had a fantastic dress. I got into the car and into the church. It all felt very vague, I thought: 'Oh my God, I hope I'm not sick.' But I was OK. I controlled myself. We then had to go to the reception, which was eight miles away, and halfway down in the taxi I had to stop and be sick.

When we got to the reception the starter was minestrone soup or melon. It was the smell of the minestrone soup that did it. I was laid out in a room and I missed the wedding meal. It really was terrible, absolutely dreadful. My daughter says: 'Oh, I had a good wedding' and I say: 'Was it good?' It was dreadful for me!

I read about feverfew in one of my daughter's magazines. I thought: 'I'll try that – in pill form.' I gave them three months and I've found that they certainly do help. I only started to notice a difference after I'd been on them three months. I take them every morning and I've been taking them for a year now. I still get migraines but I can control them better. I'm sick less. It's not quite so bad as it was before and I can usually keep going. It makes a difference.

Homoeopathy

The word *homoeo* is Greek and it means 'like'. Homoeopathy is the practice of treating like with like. Not such an extraordinary view when you consider the theory of the 'hair of the dog' or vaccinations and inoculations, where you are given a little bit of the very thing you do not want to get!

Homoeopathy was invented in the eighteenth century by a doctor called Samuel Hahnemann. He felt that traditional medicine was big on shortcomings and he believed that human beings had a capacity for healing themselves. The symptoms of a disease, he thought, were a reflection of a person's struggle to overcome harmful forces; the doctor's work should be to discover, and if possible remove, the cause of the problem and to stimulate the vital healing force of nature. Dr Hahnemann and his followers carried out experiments upon themselves. Over long periods they took small doses of poisonous or medicinal substances, carefully noting the symptoms they produced (these experiments were called Provings). Patients suffering from similar symptoms were then treated with these substances, with good results. The next step was to establish the smallest effective dose in order to avoid side-effects. To his amazement Hahnemann found that, using a special method of dilution, the more the similar remedy was diluted, the more active it became. He called this method potentization. However this paradox – that less of a substance could be more effective – was not at all acceptable to scientific thought at the time. Hahnemann and his followers were ridiculed.

Today, homoeopathy is a much respected and widely used form of medical treatment that reports good results with migraine patients. The principles are still those established by Hahnemann: the patient is treated – not the disease. So the doctor aims to get a multidimensional picture of the patient. Along with the symptoms of the illness and medical history, the doctor will want to know about the patient's personality. Is he or she quick-tempered or laid back, artistic, musical or technically minded? Does he or she like the sea or mountains? Are they happier in cold or hot weather? What is their complexion like – dark or fair, greasy or dry-skinned? Answers to questions like this help the doctor to find the remedy to match the person. So if your experience with homoeopathy has been limited to buying a remedy marked 'suitable for migraine' at the health shop or pharmacist's, you can see why it may not have worked. Off-the-shelf remedies can work for some people, but if you want to give homoeopathy a serious try it's best to see a homoeo-pathic doctor.

As far as the remedies are concerned, these are prepared from animal, vegetable and mineral sources. They are diluted, using the process of potentization that Hahnemann discovered, so that the patient receives an infinitesimal dose of the remedy which, paradox-ically, achieves the maximum effect.

The British Homoeopathic Association can give you more infor-mation on this treatment and holds a register of homoeopathic doc-tors. Some GPs practise it in their surgeries, and there are hospitals in various parts of the country that offer homoeopathy on the NHS (see Useful Addresses).

Hypnosis

This form of therapy is particularly well suited to migraine, say the practitioners. The basic aim is to shift the patient's senses from external to internal awareness so that they can look at the world inside their heads. It may sound complex, but apparently there are many techniques for achieving this and it does not take very long.

Although hypnotherapists do not claim to cure their migraine patients, they say that many do get complete and lasting relief and almost all are helped to some extent. Stephen Brooks, a senior tutor with British Hypnosis Research (a respected body of qualified prac-titioners), explains the process:

First of all we have to identify whether it is an organic problem or whether it is stress-related. If it is stress-related it is easier to help with hypnosis and psychotherapy. So we would attempt to find out what was causing it rather than tackle the symptoms alone. This may involve finding out about the patient's lifestyle, what causes them stress, traumatic events in their life and so on.

If we are able to discover that there are areas which are stress-related we will attempt first of all to change that. This may be by getting them to slow down various areas of their life or change their situation. But you have to bear in mind that often stress-related problems are there because the patient can't solve them themselves. Just telling them to do something isn't much good. You have to get in there and work psychotherapeutically with them. This can be a combination of asking patients things at a conscious level and asking them at a subconscious level because often people know things they don't know they know.

After we've taken the patient's history to identify what areas might be encouraging the problem, if we can't find anything that's somehow making it happen, we would attempt to teach the patient some sort of self-hypnosis. This is so that they can control it themselves either when it comes on or, ideally, when it is not there at all as a way of preventing it from occurring.

One technique taught is visualization. There are many different ways of teaching this, but here's an example explained by Stephen Brooks:

You can have somebody mentally going downstairs to somewhere very comfortable and relaxing – somewhere very safe and secure. Or you can take them to some very special place that they are familiar with like a holiday destination that makes them feel very good – somewhere they are normally free from the problem, so that it is a kind of mental holiday for them. This is just as a means of relaxing, and secondly to look at the physiological aspect of the problem. Most people can imagine where the pain and suffering is and, similar to the way in which people approach cancer, you actually imagine the part of you that's injured or is in pain and you use your imagination as a means of reducing the severity.

For example, if the pain is a stabbing pain it seems to suggest that it is sharp, so you could visually put soft cushions around it. Also, if it is stabbing it is not continuous, so we would attempt to use time distortion. Say, for instance, you are watching a two-hour film. If the film is interesting the two hours will seem very short. If it is boring that same time will seem very long. Your perception of time can change. We can induce time distortion with hypnosis so, for instance, a migraine attack that lasts for four hours can seem like it lasted for half an hour. In addition to that, if the pain is on-and-off we can make the periods of comfort longer and the periods of pain shorter.

The way that our practitioners work is that they are taught to do what we call 'brief therapy'. They don't spend months and years with patients in therapy. The emphasis is on giving the patient the skills or tools that they can apply themselves so that they don't become dependent. That is a very important part of what we teach. How long they are in treatment depends on the severity of the problem, the cause of the problem and the willingness of the patient to practise what they learn. On average it could be anything between one session and a dozen at the most. If someone needs a dozen sessions it usually means that their life is very complex in other areas, and a lot of investigations have to be carried out into relationships and all kinds of things like that.

If you are interested in trying hypnotherapy it is of paramount importance to find a skilled and qualified practitioner. British Hypnosis Research keeps a register of their trained hypnotherapists and weekend courses are also available.

Osteopathy

This is the science of human mechanics. The osteopath is concerned with the body framework (the musculo-skeletal system) and how it is functioning. The musculo-skeletal system is the largest system in the body, consisting primarily of the bones, joints, muscles, ligaments and connective tissue. It is the largest user of energy in the body as well as the largest producer of waste products.

It is the osteopath's job to diagnose and treat faults that occur in the body framework. These can be due to injury, stress or any other cause, and it is his or her job to make sure that it is functioning as efficiently as possible. Although backache is the most common complaint treated by osteopaths, many other conditions which affect the body frame can come into the osteopath's orbit. Headaches and neck and shoulder tension can be treated, as well as joint strains.

At the first consultation with a registered osteopath he or she will want to know how the symptoms began and the factors which affect them. A medical history will be taken and current treatment will be noted. X-rays, blood tests and/or urine analyses may also be requested. The osteopath will assess the patient's posture and structural state and make a detailed examination by touch. He will feel the range and quality of movement of the joints to note whether the movement is restricted or excessive. The condition of the soft tissues, the muscles, ligaments and connective tissues will be examined to see whether they are normal or under stress.

A variety of treatment methods may be used, ranging from soft tissue 'massage' types of technique and passive repetitive stretching movements to improve joint mobility, to the high velocity thrust technique which can cause a joint to click. Gentle release techniques are often used, particularly when treating the very young or elderly patients. Treatment can include advice on posture, diet, lifestyle or stress, since any of these may have contributed to the problem.

Do be sure to find a trained and qualified osteopath. Your doctor may be able to refer you to one. If not, find a registered osteopath who will have the letters MRO (Member of the Register of Osteopaths) after his or her name. Look under 'Osteopaths' in the Yellow Pages or other directories available at the public library.

Paula is a young working mother with a small baby. She has been suffering migraines for several years now and they have been really getting her down. But she is optimistic that she may at last be on the right track for treating them.

Paula

I get a pounding headache behind my eyes. It's there all the time. Sometimes I get what's called a blockage. I feel slightly dizzy and sick and the pain is really bad. When it's not severe I can sleep through it. When it's bad I can't. This has been going on for seven or eight years. I get depressed. It gets me down quite a bit. When it started I didn't go to the doctor for some time because I thought it was just the normal type of headache and I didn't take much notice.

I saw a neurologist and a mental health chap who gave out he couldn't understand what was wrong width me. I saw him for about two years. I had stress therapy with him. I didn't think it was stress then, and I still don't think it is. I had the migraines right through pregnancy.

The worst part was the stage when nobody seemed to be helping. The doctor suggested I go to see an acupuncturist who is a friend of his. It helped for a while, but it wasn't long-term. But now he's working together with this osteopath chap. The acupuncturist is doing the muscle relaxant and the osteopath is doing the other work. I've been going to the acupuncturist for so long that now he is treating me free of charge.

The osteopath chap said he'd treated another lady with migraine. She'd slipped over on some ice about the same time as they started happening. He's treated her back and her migraines have disappeared completely. The thing is I also slipped on some ice when I was about sixteen or seventeen which could be around the same time as the migraines started. I could have done the same – I could have hurt myself, couldn't I? The osteopath said that the side of my skull looks as if somebody had hit it with a cricket ball. All the muscles down one side are damaged.

I went to see him tonight, and it might sound funny but he drained the fluid out from my brain. I had to lie down on the bed and he supported my head and he was pressing down on my neck and drained all the fluid down. I had to lie very still and relax for about ten minutes. He pushed the little bone at the base of the spine. I could feel this fluid going bubbling down. I feel so much better now. While I was lying there it felt as if I was just floating. Now it's a fuzzy pain. But things are changing. I think I will be better.

Reflexology

This is a process based on applying pressure to minute points in the feet. Each zone of the foot correlates to a different part of the body – limbs as well as internal organs. By applying pressure on the soles of the feet it is thought that stress-related illnesses like migraine can be helped. This may come about, it is thought, by releasing endorphins – morphine-like chemicals in the brain. Also, if the patient feels pain when the therapist is massaging a certain zone in the foot, it may reveal problems in the correlating part of the body. It is a very relaxing and soothing treatment and can, of course, have therapeutic effects as well.

Relaxation therapy

Over and over again, sufferers describe the feelings of anxiety or panic they experience when they know that a major migraine attack is on the way. This feeling of impending doom or even horror can aggravate the attack, making it more severe or longer-lasting. Furthermore, the fear of an attack can often precipitate one. The last thing April wanted on her daughter's wedding day was migraine (see p. 129); yet she got 'one of the worst attacks ever.' Others of us don't get a migraine on the day we most dread getting one, but we pay for it with the mother and father of attacks the day after – when the tension and stress are over. If we could reverse the procedure and instead of getting worked up at the prospect of an attack, slow down and relax, we should be able take the edge off the attack and – who knows – maybe walk away from it altogether. The late Jane Madders pioneered relaxation techniques which she taught to fellow migraine sufferers at the Birmingham Migraine Clinic as well as at National Childbirth Trust classes. A trained PE teacher and physiotherapist, she was also one of the founder members of the Relaxation for Living charity and a friend of the Migraine Action Association.

Jane's methods involve a simple form of muscle control, learnt as a physical skill and then applied to daily living situations. She explained: 'It involves the recognition of unnecessary and inappropriate muscle tension and how to release it and then to apply it everyday situations. There is evidence that when you are relaxed you begin to feel peaceful and rested and the message gets to your body that there is no need to be prepared for fight or flight and the churning dies down.

To relax, you must first be aware of tension. Sitting down can hard work. Jane said:

> Your shoulders may be held tight so that the muscles may even have gone into cramp-like spasm causing the tender spots so familiar to tense people. Your teeth may be clenched producing a ridge of hard muscle by your temples, your abdominal muscles held in so tightly that your stomach aches with the effort. Your forehead may be strained, your hands tense. All this is using as much energy as if you were doing hard work. In this sustained tension, which may go on all day, there is little opportunity for the clearing away of fatigue waste products in the bloodstream as there is in rhythmical movement. It is hardly surprising that you are tired at the end of the day and your muscles ache, especially those of the neck and shoulders.

Jane's techniques, which are taught by Relaxation for Living, involve learning to recognize tense muscles and how to relax them. Relaxation for Living have qualified teachers who run group classes throughout the country. The classes last about two hours each and you are given a series of simple exercises to practise at home as well as on your way to work – for instance, sitting at the wheel of a car in a traffic jam. The idea is to incorporate these techniques into your daily life. The course covers the use of relaxation techniques for particular conditions like migraine and insomnia.

In addition to the practical exercises the course covers the theory of stress management, and the lesson ends with a group discussion. The classes are not expensive. Correspondence courses, cassette tapes and publications on the subject are also available from Relaxation for Living (see Useful Addresses).

Traditional Chinese medicine

This is very different in concept from traditional Western medicine. Chinese medicine not only looks at the symptoms of the disease but it also takes into account the age, habits, physical and emotional aspects of the individual. It tries to get a picture of the patient in order to evaluate any patterns of disharmony that have arisen. Chinese medicine believes that health is a state of total harmony between the physical, emotional and spiritual aspects of the individual. Illness, on the other hand, is a disharmony that manifests itself as certain symptoms. The symptoms on their own are often unimportant, and are merely part of the harmony or disharmony which makes up the whole person.

The Chinese doctor will notice the patient's posture, the way he or she moves, the complexion, brightness of the eyes and so on. But most important to the diagnosis is the state of the patient's tongue. The theory is that the tongue connects to every meridian, channel and organ in the body and so the quality of its coating, colour, size, shape and movement all have a bearing on the state of the internal organs.

The quality of the patient's voice and his manner of speaking are noted, as are bodily odours. The patient is, of course, asked to describe symptoms, and he or she will be asked questions related to urination, bowel function, sleep patterns, feelings of cold, heat, unusual thirst, funny taste in the mouth and so on, much the same way as in Western medicine. The pulse is felt at the wrists on the radial artery; its strength, rhythm and quality indicate the balance of energy and the state of the disease. When a diagnosis is made, the doctor will prescribe herbs, acupuncture, massage or meditation or maybe a combination.

Chinese medicine has proved effective at treating eczema in both children and adults. Doctors at Great Ormond Street Hospital for Sick Children saw remarkable cures in severe cases of eczema which they had previously been unable to treat. Currently, traditional Chinese medicine is being researched in British hospitals for its efficacy in treating asthma, psoriasis and migraine.

Transcendental meditation

Many people – including six hundred doctors in the UK – practise meditation to control stress and, in so doing, to promote energy and good health. There are many different techniques you can learn, of which one of the easiest and most readily available is transcendental meditation – the one that the Beatles made famous all those years ago. A great deal of research has gone into TM since then and it seems that many of the claims made by TM's inventor, Maharishi Mahesh Yogi, and his followers are not unfounded. A large insurance company in Holland now offers a 30 per cent discount on life insurance policies to TM meditators!

The technique is not at all difficult to master. In a one-to-one session you are given a special sound or phrase called a mantra. You shut your eyes, quieten your thoughts and focus on the mantra. This helps get rid of all the little jumbled ideas that race across your mind. Eventually you let go of the mantra and achieve a deep sense of stillness and inner quiet. The meditating sessions last between fifteen and twenty minutes, but the feeling of peace stays with you, to some extent, throughout the day. As you become a regular meditator – and you are supposed to do it twice a day – this inner peaceful feeling is constantly replenished and emphasized. It is as simple as that.

For a stress-related illness like migraine, meditation has a very special place. Research has discovered that, while sleep triggers the body's restorative powers, the deeper state of mental relaxation achieved during meditation allows this repair work and recuperation to be carried out more efficiently. It can also help alleviate accumulated stress and the illnesses that this build-up of stress can cause.

Learning the technique doesn't come cheap but it is a one-off payment that lasts for life – subsequent check-ups, if you need them, are free. It is a seven-stage course which you can learn in about a week.

Yoga

Not so much a therapy, more a way of life, yoga is a system of mental, physical and spiritual development which originated in India some three thousand years ago. It can be practised by anyone at any age.

As far as the migraine sufferer is concerned, it can certainly help by putting the body into as good a working condition as it can achieve and teaching both mind and body to let go and relax. After a while this feeling of relaxation remains with you when you leave the classroom or when you finish the practice session and helps you sleep at night. But first you have to learn and you have to practise.

The British Wheel of Yoga says:

In repose, muscles constantly receive messages from the nervous system, keeping them in a constant state of slight contraction. This muscle 'tonus' is what keeps the body together and enables it to move. Tonus varies according to whether we are awake or asleep. Certain muscles are more controlled than others and their tone is also affected by our emotional state. Each thought or emotional change alters the level of muscle tension, but those who live in a constant state of anxiety will have a high level of muscle tension, being continually stretched tight as a drum.

Relaxation is as much mental as physical. In order to keep a balanced level of tension there must be harmony between body and mind. Our thoughts reflect our physical state and vice versa. The key to this state of harmony, according to Yoga teachings, is the breath. When anxiety and muscle tension are high, breathing is short and centred around the upper chest. When energy is low, particularly after prolonged illness or depression, breathing is centred around the diaphragm and rarely reaches the upper chest.

By changing the way we breathe and learning to make full use of the lungs, we can change the way we feel and energy resources are increased as the bloodstream receives a richer supply of oxygen and heart and lungs are strengthened. Students who learn to relax properly often speak of an increased feeling of well-being and vitality.

In a yoga class you will start by learning a series of stretching exercises to enable the body to become more supple. The emphasis in yoga is very much on individual development. The fact that someone else in the class may be able to contort their body into a figure of eight is of no relevance to you. Some yoga teachers ask their class to keep their eyes closed while doing the asanas (yoga postures), both to increase concentration and to bring home the non-competitive nature of the exercise. You will also learn breathing techniques. The classes almost invariably finish with a period of relaxation, when students are taught how to direct the mind to different parts of the body and instruct it to relax. This is followed by ten minutes or so of deep relaxation.

Meditation is of course a very important part of the yoga teaching. Different methods are used to quieten or concentrate the mind so as to achieve an inner silence. The meditation may involve the use of a visual object (the 'sight' technique) or of sound as in a mantra, which forms the basis of transcendental meditation (see p. 127). Another form of yoga meditation uses the technique of concentrating on the breath.

If you are interested in taking up yoga you would be well advised to go to a class given by a qualified teacher. Most of the postures take a certain amount of learning and it is important to get them right – you cannot be sure of doing this from a book or video, though these can be useful once you have got into the swing of yoga. Group classes are not usually expensive and they can be quite social. The British Wheel of Yoga have qualified teachers who run classes throughout the country.

14

The Migraine Action Association (formerly the British Migraine Association)

The founder – Peter Wilson MBE

The story of the founding of the British Migraine Association is very much the story of one man – a sufferer whose migraines nearly cost him his life. In the winter of 1943 Peter Wilson was on board a Royal Navy ship, escorting a wartime convoy between Murmansk in northern Russia and Scapa Flow in the Orkneys. Peter was on watch. He began to tell the story in a book which he had just started writing before he died; in fact only two chapters were written.

At the very crack of dawn, all heavens broke loose upon us as a 152 mph hurricane struck right out of the blue with the most terrifying force of shrieking winds and huge black mountainous waves. We were being treated to the privilege of witnessing one of Mother Nature's rarest spectacles of her most awful fury. All day and into the night the hurricane raged on, the huge cresting rollers sweeping our decks clean from stern post to stern in boiling anger.

Exhausted and exhilarated came the moment of truth for me as every bedevilled ingredient compounded into the most classical of classical migraines. As the warning bells rang out loud and clear I struggled through a four-hour watch of urgent deciphering, my head throbbing into increasing agonies as the inexorable progress of the attack developed.

By middle watch I was relieved duties and despite the strictest order for all but the bridge duty men to stay below, I staggered upwards on to the seething quarterdeck to gasp in great gulps of ice fresh air. Almost immediately a huge wave swept inboard, washing me straight over the side into the black hell of no return. No moment of grace to contemplate the sudden ending of a life of so little consequence – just a numbed terror freezing into my whole wretched being. And then, so strangely, overlaying all despair, the shattering pain and bitter anger against my inherited enemy.

As the ship dropped like a stone into the valley of a mountainous wave, came a momentary calm and with it, the miracle of reprieve to live another day. I was tossed back almost to the door from which I had so suddenly made an exit. I came to at the foot of a steep ladder from which I had fallen in my desperation. I was kept in the sick bay for twelve hours when, having completed the course of puking indignities, I was able to contemplate my good fortune. All was peace again. The hammering devils had retreated to return another day in less dramatic circumstances. But the seed of my revenge had now been deeply sown.

But it was a good fifteen years before Peter was to have revenge on his 'inherited enemy' with the founding of the British Migraine Association. He knew about migraine from his childhood, and recalled:

My very first memories of the wretchedness of the condition I was to inherit were of my mother writhing in agony with vinegar-soaked compresses on her forehead and emptied packets of the then famous Daisy Powders preceding the more common aspirins of today. Since my mother invariably made a perfect recovery within hours and everyone tip-toed around the house in order not to disturb her sleeping, I hardly realized the full impact of domestic upset occasioned by the absence of the mainspring of every household.

As to my own sufferings, these were not to start in earnest until I was twelve years of age, but the memory of that first attack is as clear sixty-five years later as it was the evening I arrived at our Scout campsite in South Devon when I really thought I must be dying. Travel sickness appeared to be the problem at that stage and many millions of sufferers will have shared so many agonizing holiday journeys ruining so many happy family trips.

Although I also have everlasting memories of so many holiday journeys ending in agony and distress, the truly recurring attacks only started after I was married at the age of twenty-four. My career suffered as the frequency of attacks grew. It is the absurd speed between perfect normality and sudden collapse into writhing prostration which offers the greatest offence to the rest of the family, friends or employers. And the sickening thoughts of inferiority surge like waves as an extra mental burden.

Early in 1958, now working in the Corporation Treasurer's Department in Bournemouth (where he remained for twenty-five years) Peter went to buy some aspirins at Boots. While he was there he told the chemist, George Bell, of his determination to do something one day to help other migraine sufferers. George, a migraine sufferer himself, encouraged him. By sheer coincidence, this same year Peter experienced a remission from his migraine attacks which lasted a few years.

Peter spent his savings on the printing of his first leaflet on migraine, and placed an advertisement in the *Bournemouth Evening Echo* inviting sufferers to meet him at a fellow sufferer's flat. Nine turned up – George Bell being among them. Each of them, including Peter, put £10 into the kitty and formed the British Migraine Association; Peter was elected its Hon. Secretary.

From this point on, Peter began in earnest his campaign to get something done. He realized, right from the start, that if the Association was to get off the ground he would have to capture the interest of leading opinion formers as well as the medical world. He put his next advertisement in the *Daily Telegraph*. It resulted in the recruitment of one Nobel Prize winner, four well-known writers, two famous scientists, a number of doctors and a hundred other people. They were the start of a membership which, at Peter's death in 1987, totalled over seven thousand. Working from home, in his spare time, Peter organized a series of medical symposia. He explained:

> Probably the most productive occasions during our early stages were the intimate weekend discussions we arranged for those specialists we knew to have a special interest in migraine. Held at various Bournemouth hotels a select group of doctors were invited with their wives – allowing a little light social atmosphere but where doctors were able to discuss, far into the night, in extended argument. It was research funds well spent and the high quality of relaxed interchange of experience and argued reasoning reflected great credit on the Association's motives and acceptability of what might have been seen as a purely 'consumer' outlook. These weekends were organized as frequently as we could afford and very soon an extremely formidable team of the most dedicated experts emerged to spread the freshening interest throughout the world. We had created an awakening.

But it was not all plain sailing.

> Not all of our plans reached full fruition. Our very first project to be agreed by our medical advisory team was the well-planned clinical trial of a well-established drug used in the prophylactic treatment of migraine. Ten general practitioners, all members of the Royal College of GPs, who were fairly well distributed over the

UK, were to undertake their own assessments of the drug on their migraine patients and to send their monthly observations to the selected co-ordinator – a doctor of the highest reliability who had written an excellent paper on the value of the drug. The whole idea was based on his own suggestion.

It was to be a model trial with every safeguard duly inserted and we all had the highest hopes for a most successful outcome – a blueprint for all future trials. The months passed by but when I enquired how matters were developing, it transpired that the doctor chosen to assemble all the reports had simply ignored them and had retired into the depths of Cornwall never to be heard of again. My first taste of broken faith in human nature at the Top. Alas, by no means an isolated disappointment but all part of the hardening process so inevitable in an imperfect world.

None the less Peter battled on, aided by his wife, Peggy – who was not a migraine sufferer. The Association received support and help from drug manufacturers.

In 1962 Bayer Products sponsored a most generous weekend symposium on our behalf at the Mount Royal Hotel in London where we welcomed 250 doctors and their wives. A massive extension of our more intimate weekend discussions but reaching through to the GPs as well as the consultants. And it was thanks to Sandoz Ltd that we were able to equip our very own Migraine Clinic and Institute in Bournemouth, under the direction of Dr Vera Walker, consultant at the Oxford Eye Hospital and an acknowledged world authority on allergy. With the support of many of our members we were able to rent and furnish the flat above our office where Dr Walker was able to treat, advise and refer to other specialists so many of our members in the most relaxed circumstances.

The British Migraine Association changed its name in 1997 to the Migraine Action Association and under that name continues to pursue strong ties with the drug companies.

The fates that allowed Peter remission from his migraines and the confidence with which to forge ahead with establishing the new Association must have felt that they had been kind for long enough. Peter wrote:

At this stage my own attacks started again, sparked no doubt by the endless hours hunched over a hot typewriter, often into the small hours in order to keep pace with the avalanche of letters calling for individual thought and caring. It was probably good for my soul and at least I now had my own techniques and antidotes for speedier relief – not always effective though and then the subsequent horrors of total prostration for the twenty-four hours I could not afford to lose.

The Migraine Trust

The medical meetings and weekends continued, and the Association sponsored awards for essays and research papers in general practice. Then came the next step.

In one of the medical gatherings the decision was agreed by the senior doctors present that Lord Brain – the leading authority in world neurology be asked to head the formation of a strictly medical organization for the study and research into migraine. The fact that such an eminent world figure should wholeheartedly believe that it was time for such a learned society to be launched proved beyond all doubt that we had been completely justified in our campaigning. Dr Robert Smith from the Wellcome Foundation was asked to start laying the foundations for what was later to be known as the Migraine Trust – a title which Lord Brain had asked me to decide upon – with the alternative of Headache Foundation and other possible titles.

Now began the most frantic series of evening meetings held at the Wellcome Foundation and most generously sponsored by Wellcome. Lord (C.P.) Snow and Lady Snow (the authoress Pamela Hansford-Johnson) were asked to bring their brilliant intellects into play and our Hon.Treasurer and I were also asked to submit our own ideas for the constitution of the Trust. Senior consultants, city VIPs and representatives of the Ministry of Health joined us at these exciting evening gatherings and slowly the new body took shape. The Association footed the bill for the legal charges and the initial public relations campaign brought in to launch the official appeal to industry, commerce and the City of London interests.

It was left to Dr Smith and myself to search for office premises and liaise with the PR company. Broadcasts were made and slowly the essential funds accrued. The first thousand pounds was a sum the Association had reserved against such a day and which had been donated to us by Lord Snow.

In 1966 the Migraine Trust was formed, under the chairmanship of Lord Brain, with the British Migraine Association donating £3300 towards the initial costs. Peter was invited to accept the office of

Director to the Trust but felt unable to take it on since he would have had either to move to London or commute daily from Bournemouth. He wrote:

> Although a Londoner by birth I had no strong desire to return to the hassle of teeming life in the capital, particularly as I was now happily settled in my work at the Town Hall and my cosy office at home where I could stare out over my neighbours' gardens to my heart's content whenever inspiration failed me. Cursed with an untidy mind I felt free to scatter papers and notes with total abandon.

But as a member of the Trust's management committee, he was still very involved with getting the Trust up and running.

> The exciting business of weaning the Trust into healthy stature became tightly interwoven with the Association's own work – the endless composition of letters to be dealt with, each one completely individual and requiring a simple sincerity and deep understanding. Then there was the writing of our newsletter which had to reflect faith, hope and charity – no easy task to an ill-equipped intellect of my lowly status. It was a question of long periods of blankness trying to squeeze the right words from a very spongey mind. Time was of the essence since I felt compelled to reply by return of post to almost everything. Burning the midnight oil was my one defence.
>
> Events were now happening thick and fast. A prestigious office was found in Queen Square in London and a retired Naval Captain engaged to open fire as the first Director of the Trust. His first duties were directed to working with an experienced public relations company in approaching the city merchants for financial support. An imposing list of many famous names was assembled and it is doubtful whether any organization has seen such an array of eminent supporters.

One such supporter was Sir Barnes Wallis of bouncing bomb fame who was a lifelong migraine sufferer.

In 1970 the Trust, supported financially by donations from the British Migraine Association and other funds, was able to found a migraine clinic in the City of London. Princess Margaret (a migraine sufferer herself) opened it and gave her name to it.

Peter's efforts were officially recognized when in 1967 he was awarded an MBE. This was a remarkable achievement for anyone, let alone a man with no medical qualifications or contacts in the corridors of power.

In May 1987 Peter suffered a stroke and died shortly afterwards. He is remembered by friends, colleagues and associates as a clever, kind, funny man, who always proffered a shoulder to cry on but seldom spoke of his own health problems. His twenty-four-hour migraine attacks were severe and very painful and he would get very sick. 'The pain of migraine is so terrible,' he said, undoubtedly from personal experience, 'there is the indignity of it and then the constant fear of the next attack. And it is so humiliating when people say dismissively: "Oh, he's got another of his bloody headaches." ' Peter Wilson made sure that a lot of very important and powerful people took his 'bloody headaches' and those of millions of fellow sufferers seriously.

Jo Liddell – director

Whether or not there is such a thing as a migraine personality is still very much a question of conjecture, but what seems to be far more certain is that along with the migraines comes the fighting spirit. And this spirit is very much encapsulated in the personality of Jo Liddell, who took over from Peter in 1981. Over the past decade Jo's name has become synonymous with migraine both amongst sufferers and in the medical world. She is the migraine help-line, answering numerous phone calls and letters every day. Like Peter, she answers each letter individually, and in fact she still writes to some of his regular correspondents.

Jo speaks at meetings and conferences all over the world. She gives interviews to newspapers, radio and television and champions the cause of sufferers by writing articles on migraine for the medical press. The membership of the British Migraine Association in 1981 was three thousand; today it totals more than ten thousand. But perhaps the hallmark of her personality can be highlighted in a little anecdote.

Jo was chatting to a prominent neurologist at a meeting when she noticed that one of the members sitting nearby was looking very tearful and green about the gills. She went straight over and discovered, as she suspected, that the lady was in the throes of an unexpected migraine attack. Jo sat with the sufferer and talked to her, discovering that she took Migraleve but had forgotten to bring it with her. Jo found someone else who had some, organized a glass of water and a biscuit, and stayed with the lady until she felt confident that she was going to be all right. Like Peter, Jo has never lost sight of what it's all about.

Like Peter, Jo grew up in a migraine household. Her mother suffered with migraine and, similarly, Jo had it as a child. But unlike Peter's, Jo's migraines did not spontaneously remit. She suffered very severe attacks, sometimes lasting three to five days each, and they often came as frequently as twice a month. So she spent almost as much time with a migraine as without one. To get over this unacceptable state of affairs she had to find a solution – something that would work for her. Here's her story:

I remember my first migraine. I was about eight. It was just after Christmas and we were taken to see the film of Treasure Island as a treat. I don't remember anything about the film, but I remember vividly afterwards, lying in bed in the dark, listening to the sounds of everyone having tea. My mother came to see how I was feeling and she tells me that I said: 'If only you could cut my head down the middle and take half of it away, I would be all right'– and she thought: 'Poor little scrap, she's got it too.'

My mother's migraine had more effect on me than my own attacks in my childhood and in my teens. Mine were not too bad at that time – not very frequent and not too severe – and a few hours' sleep could make me well again. My mother's migraine was in a different league altogether. One of the worst things was that, in those days, no one understood what was really the matter with her. Yes, she had severe migraine headaches, but what were the other strange symptoms? Jumbled-up words, partial paralysis, even temporary blindness. She was prescribed various drugs, mainly sedatives, which made her feel awful, but we were so frightened we encouraged her to persevere with them. Eventually she was prescribed ergotamine, but was not given the right advice on its use. She hated taking drugs so much that she would delay taking the ergotamine, hoping that this time it would not be a bad attack and, of course, if ergotamine is not taken really early in an attack it is of very little use.

My own migraines were comparatively easy to manage in my teens and early twenties. A doctor gave me some good advice. She said that if three aspirins did not relieve my pain then aspirin was not the right drug for me. She also said that people like me should eat 'little and often'. I switched my painkillers to compound codeine and took care not to go too long without food. During the war I did not eat my sweet ration for pleasure, but kept it for emergencies. All the things that could happen in those days that could delay a meal were an extra hazard for me. But forewarned is forearmed and I usually coped.

While clothes were rationed, a cousin of mine gave me one of her frocks, a beautiful dress with a pleated skirt. Unfortunately it was in navy and white striped linen. Neither my mother nor I could iron it without triggering a migraine, and sadly I gave it away.

Other life choices were affected by my migraines. I certainly chose my husband for his kindness and understanding as well as for his other sterling qualities. We had an extremely simple wedding. I had heard about my mother's nightmare 'big' wedding when she had a dreadful migraine all day and I didn't want history to be repeated, for me or for her.

Migraine became a serious problem for me in my mid-thirties. I was more or less free from attacks during the five years or so that I was having my children, but migraine returned and the demands of bringing up three lively children plus a part-time teaching job meant that it became urgent that I find some help. Like many migraine sufferers, I was convinced that what I really needed was a very strong painkiller, but all my doctor prescribed was yet another version of the sort of painkillers that I could buy for myself over the counter. One day I was prescribed ergotamine, but I found that it made me very sick – even the smell of the tablet set my stomach churning. Back to the doctor once more, and this time he prescribed ergotamine in suppository form.

I was about to go and live in America for a year and the ergotamine certainly helped me, but it was socially very inconvenient to take. One day, in the USA, when I was recovering from a three-day migraine, I met a doctor friend and his wife. I must have been looking ill, because she asked her husband if he could do anything for me. This doctor wrote out a prescription for an ergotamine inhaler. I found that it was also available in England when I returned and it kept me going nicely for about ten years.

Then ergotamine seemed to stop working for me – I was having more and more three-day migraines and I began to be horribly sick every time. I suspected that it might be the result of too much ergotamine and decided to stop using it. Then it was back to floundering around, at least two big migraines a month, plus some threatened ones and other kinds of headaches most of the rest of the time. I decided to make a very determined effort to improve things. I systematically eliminated certain foods from my diet – no difference. I went to a local GP who was an acupuncturist – that made me worse but we parted friends. I went to see a very well-known 'hormone' man who did his best to help me, but once again this made my migraines worse. Another doctor friend gave me some sample packs of Migraleve about this time and, if taken early enough, these definitely seemed to prevent some migraine attacks from developing fully.

One day, after a particularly bad bout, our solicitor phoned about something. When he heard that I was recovering from a migraine he told me that he had just read in the local paper that the British Migraine Association was holding a coffee evening that night. He came round and drove me there – I was not in a fit state to drive myself. I was

amazed to find all these pleasant people, who seemed to really under-
stand my problems, and decided to join them. I soon became the chair-
man of the local group and got to know Peter Wilson.

During all this time I had been doing full-time teaching at our local
college of education. Most of my migraines seemed to come at weekends
and, although I was often at the 'walking wounded' stage of a migraine
while at college, I managed to do a good job. I don't think that my
students ever suffered.

Things began to get worse again and one day I was asked to go and
see the principal. He wanted to know why I was having so many odd
days off. He hinted that perhaps I should find a less demanding job. So
I went back to see my GP. To my surprise I found that my old doctor had
died and a new young man was behind his desk. I told him my story and
showed him my diary with all the mig-days marked. He prescribed a
long-term preventative drug and to my amazement told me to go back
to him in a month and tell him how I got on. One month later I went
joyfully back to tell him that, although I was getting just as many
migraines, they were not so severe and they didn't last so long. I was
very pleased. He amazed me again by saying: 'We can do better than
that.' He prescribed a different kind of long-term drug and my life was
utterly changed. My migraines just stopped. It took a while to believe it
and it took even longer for my husband and family to realize that this
new woman could gad about, making up for lost time.

Soon after this I became Secretary of the British Migraine
Association and I now know that my experiences with migraine are
echoed all over the world. I have been lucky that the long-term preven-
tatives work for me, they do not have the same effect on everyone and
some people have conditions that contra-indicate their use.

No one likes to take drugs all the time, but my daily pill has kept me
on my feet for nine years now. Some migraines break through nowa-
days, but they are never as long, strong or as bad as they used to be.

'Making up for lost time' has certainly been Jo's credo over the
past ten years, and migraine sufferers have reaped the benefit of her
energies. Among the achievements that have given her the most sat-
isfaction she cites increased awareness of migraine in the media and,
as a result, in the population as a whole. 'When I began as Hon.
Secretary the press cutting service used to send us a small envelope
of cuttings about once a month,' she recalls. 'Now we get two fat
envelopes of cuttings sometimes twice a week.' Migraine is very
much in the consciousness of the medical world and lay people
worldwide, and both Peter Wilson and Jo Liddell have been responsible for putting it there.

What the Migraine Action Association Does

Since its inception in 1958, the aims of the Association have stayed the same:

- To encourage and support research into migraine.
- To gather and pass on information about drugs and treatments available for the control and relief of migraine.
- To provide friendly, cheerful reassurance and understanding with encouragement to fight back by supporting research.

The Association aims to bridge the gap between the sufferer and the medical world. To do this they publish leaflets, answer members' letters and phone calls, and produce a regular newsletter. Members can go and meet other sufferers at local groups and listen to talks, often given by leading doctors in the migraine field. In the past many members have supported research by filling in questionnaires, giving blood and urine samples, taking part in drug trials and collecting and donating considerable sums of money. The Association's leaflets and newsletters are distributed to clinics and hospital libraries throughout the country, and it is a recognized source of information for writers and broadcasters, newspapers and magazines, television and radio. Membership is worldwide, and similar associations have been set up in many other countries. In 1997, the British Migraine Association changed its name to the Migraine Action Association. If you would like to join, write for information to: The Migraine Action Association, 178a High Road, Byfleet, Surrey KT14 7ED.

15

A-Z of Migraine Tips and Triggers

In the thirty years and more since the setting up of the Migraine Action Association we have received thousands of letters and phone calls from sufferers. Along with the cries for help we have received tips and information on ways to cope with migraine. Here is a round up of the kind of information you don't always get from medical sources but is passed on from one sufferer to another. A number of triggers are included here that have not been mentioned already, as well as reminders of some of the basic rules for keeping migraine at bay.

Act quickly

Fast action when you know a migraine is on the way can prevent a full attack developing. Some patients find that painkillers plus metoclopramide at this stage can do the trick. Others find non-drug methods helpful: drinking two to three glasses of water, taking glucose tablets, and of course eating. One member swears by slices of bread. Other people say they drink coffee which at other times they avoid – some recommend extremely strong coffee. One lady takes a hot shower without a shower cap.

However, many of us get false alarms, and the last thing we want is to swallow pills on the off chance that it is a genuine attack. The best way of dealing with this situation is to get to know the pattern of your migraines intimately. Write down everything you feel or experience just before an attack is threatened. There may be certain feelings or body changes that occur before a real attack and not before a false alarm.

Once you can differentiate between a real attack and just the threat of one (or a big one as opposed to a side show) you can act quickly while your stomach is still moving. Remember that, even if you do not feel sick at first, absorption from the stomach is slowed down during an attack – so take any anti-sickness pills you may have been prescribed straightaway. Some people find soluble or effervescent tablets best, as they are more easily absorbed.

Alcohol

This can be a trigger for some sufferers, although most people can tolerate certain alcoholic drinks and not others. Red wine, port, brandy and sherry are among the worst offenders. Women suffering from menstrual migraine may well find that they can drink what they like just after their period but are much more sensitive before.

Allergies and sensitivities

The role of allergies is controversial. There is a good deal of circumstantial evidence to support the idea that some foods or chemicals can cause migraines, but little laboratory evidence. Many people find that certain foods or smells can provoke an attack, but whether this is truly an allergic reaction is open to doubt. The most commonly cited foods are:

- Cheese
- Chocolate
- Citrus fruits
- Alcohol
- Fried food
- Coffee
- Tea
- Pork
- Onions
- Sea food

If you think that food may be one of your triggers, keep a careful diary of everything you eat (remember that packets or tins of food or convenience meals may contain some of your suspected triggers). You can then look back to see what you ate in the thirty-six hours preceding a migraine; over several attacks this might give you an idea of possible causes. You can also try cutting out certain foods completely for a while to see if your attacks become less frequent.

Aspirin

Some sufferers find that taking half a soluble aspirin every day helps to prevent attacks. Doses of 300mg on alternate days have also been tried and found successful. But please don't embark on this course of treatment without checking first with your doctor. For more information on aspirin see Chapter 11.

Be prepared

Always keep your usual medicine with you so that you are not caught out. Check that you have these medicines handy whether you are going away for the day or weekend or on holiday. Don't leave home without them!

Blood sugar

Some sufferers find that going without food causes migraine attacks. This is to do with reduction in blood sugar levels. Women suffering from premenstrual migraines are likely to be particularly sensitive to low blood sugar levels during the days before their period. Normally patients should not go more than five hours without eating. Premenstrually, cut this down to no more than three hours. Small, frequent meals are better than large, irregular ones. If you don't know when you are next going to eat, have a snack – but not a chocolate or sugary one as this will cause a temporary rise in blood sugar followed by a rapid fall as the body produces insulin to cope with the sugar.

If you are dieting, consider a Weight Watchers type of diet, which includes plenty of fresh fruit, vegetables and salad as well as bread, crackers, rice and pasta – this tends to keep the blood sugar level steady. Always eat breakfast, and if your migraines follow a lie-in you may have gone without food for longer than normal. Try getting up to eat something at your normal time and then going back to bed, or have a snack by your bedside. If you are travelling or going out for the day it is worth taking a snack with you in case food is not easily available.

Breakfast

Don't skip it. Make sure you have carbohydrates and some protein Cereal with milk, for example, is fine. If your child suffers from migraine, breakfast is a must (see Chapter 8).

Caffeine

Some sufferers' attacks are less frequent or severe if they avoid caffeine, which is found most commonly in coffee, tea, chocolate cocoa and cola drinks. A naturally occurring substance in many plants, it acts as a stimulant on the central nervous system. There is no evidence to suggest that a moderate consumption harms the average healthy adult, but people's tolerance of caffeine varies according to their general health. It is generally recognized that more than 600mg per day is excessive. Some people such as pregnant women, nursing mothers and some migraine sufferers, are advised for medical reasons to cut down their caffeine intake.

Here is the caffeine content of some drinks:

	Quantity of drink (oz)	Average caffeine content (mg)
Brewed coffee	5	85
Instant coffee	5	70
Tea leaf/bag	5	40
Cocoa/hot chocolate	5	4
Coca cola	12	45
Pepsi Cola	12	38
Cola drinks	6	18

You can try cutting down or cutting them out completely for a while. One of our members who admits to being a coffee addict found that she could drink it so long as she did not take more than three different brands in a twenty-four-hour period (since her job involved visiting people she was offered a variety during the day). So she now takes her own jar of coffee from place to place. Decaffeinated tea and coffee are available, but some people find that even these can provoke attacks. If caffeine is a trigger for you, remember that it is often found in compound pain relievers, and is an ingredient of Cafergot, so you may need to switch to another tablet.

Caffeine withdrawal headaches

At the Princess Margaret Migraine Clinic case histories were taken of the daily habits of 120 weekend migraine sufferers. It was found that rising later on Saturday or Sunday mornings, coupled with a change in coffee-drinking habits, were the principal causes. A lie-in was not enough in itself to trigger an attack; the coffee factor was the clincher. People who drink large amounts of coffee during the week could be experiencing caffeine withdrawal headaches at the weekend. Those who suffer from severe headache after a general anaesthetic could be experiencing the same symptoms.

One medical theory, according to the Diamond Headache Clinic, is that, since caffeine constricts the blood vessels, continual intake may cause them to adapt to a semi-constricted state. Sudden withdrawal of caffeine can cause the vessels to dilate which produces headache. Also, since caffeine is a stimulant, when you cut down drastically or come off it you can experience 'let down' feelings.

Cheese

Cheese is thought to trigger attacks in some sufferers. The undesirable effect is thought to be due to a chemical called tyramine, which is present in most cheeses and occurs naturally in the body. One of a group of chemical compounds called amines, which are important in the working of the brain and the circulation of the blood, tyramine is known as a vasoactive amine because it has a direct action on the blood vessels. It is thought to cause both hormonal and circulatory changes in the bodies of susceptible people. Cheeses that have no detectable traces of tyramine are cottage cheese, quark, Philadelphia and curd. All the rest contain, as far as is known, some quantity of tyramine. Some people say that cooked cheese is the worst.

Chinese restaurant syndrome

This is caused by monosodium glutamate, a flavour enhancer, that is regularly added to Chinese food. The symptoms are a pain in the forehead, face and neck, often accompanied by a feeling of tightness on the face. Some people may even feel sick and dizzy, and suffer stomach pains and diarrhoea. Many other foods apart from Chinese also contain monosodium glutamate – convenience foods and soup, to name but two. If you identify this additive as a trigger you will need to look out for it (it is also sometimes called E621) on all the tinned and prepared foods that you buy. Some people are so sensitive to this substance that they can recognize the smell immediately.

Another theory is that the syndrome may be caused not by MSG but by hunger. You may not eat anything for some hours beforehand so as not to spoil your appetite for the goodies in store at the restaurant. So the migraine may be triggered by a drop in blood sugar. Next time, try eating something before you leave for the restaurant. It may save you a lot of time at the supermarket checking labels, and you won't have to give up those delicious Chinese meals!

Chocolate

This has been high on the list of possible migraine triggers for some time. Chocolate contains several amines including phenylethylamine, which is vasoactive. It also contains caffeine. However, not every sufferer is affected by chocolate, and some specialists believe that chocolate is sometimes, and for some people, wrongly branded as the culprit. A strong desire for something sweet is often a precursor to a migraine attack. So the theory goes that at that stage you reach out for a bar of chocolate. A little while later the migraine arrives, and as you think back to what you ate, the image of the chocolate looms large. But in fact the trigger, if there was a dietary one, could have been anything you ate in the previous twenty-four to thirty-six hours. To check whether you are sensitive to chocolate take yourself off it completely for a month or more. You could try carob as a substitute. Scan the contents of everything you eat to see that there is no chocolate or cocoa present. Then put yourself back on it and see what happens.

Citrus fruits

These also contain a vasoactive amine, synephrine. Concentrated fruit juice is considered to be the worst and this is probably because the whole orange, including the skin, is crushed to produce the concentrate and there are higher levels of amines in the skin than in the fruit. If you discover that this is a trigger for you, examine the contents of convenience foods and ready-made dishes for lemon or orange juice.

Cold packs

Some people find a cold pack on the head, neck and/or stomach (if nausea is present) a great relief during an attack. These are available from chemists, some camping shops or by mail order. In an emergency, just take a packet of frozen vegetables out of the freezer. One ten-year-old patient wrote to say that she puts half a pint of cold water inside a balloon and places that over the affected eye. Some sufferers prefer to use packs at hand-hot temperature.

Compresses

One sufferer wrote that she has abandoned using painkillers during her attacks, but instead uses hot and cold compresses. She has two bowls, one filled with very hot water and the other with very cold water. She soaks a cloth in the very hot water, wrings it out and places it on her forehead. She does this three times. She then repeats the process with the cold water. This, she says, gives great relief.

Contraceptive pill

Many more women than men suffer from migraine, which is thought to be the effect of hormones. Some women find that their attacks start, or become worse, when on the Pill; if this is so for you, it may be advisable to try a different brand or perhaps change to a different method of contraception. If you suspect that the Pill is affecting you, consult your doctor or family planning clinic. If the migraines started or got worse as a result of your taking the Pill they will usually get better or go once you come off it.

Dark glasses

Wearing dark glasses can help. Members who wear glasses like lenses that change with the intensity of light, especially on bright days. These can be worn indoors as well. If you think you need even darker than usual sunglasses, try sports shops for ski glasses. Get good big lenses so that light does not enter around the sides. Wide side-pieces may also help.

Dental migraines

Tooth problems can cause pain in one or both sides of the head. This is usually due to the teeth on one side being higher than on the other, which results in an asymmetrical bite. In *Understanding Headaches and Migraines* Dr J. N. Blau writes that the Migraine Action Association arranged for twenty migraine patients from the Charing Cross Hospital Migraine Clinic to be seen by a professor of dentistry at Guy's Hospital Dental School. The professor was particularly interested in this condition which is known as 'dental malocclusion'. He found that six of the 20 had abnormalities of bite. This was corrected, and one of the six reported fewer migraines.

Diary

Keep a comprehensive diary of your attacks to try and identify special triggers and any obvious pattern of attacks. Your diary should include all foods and drink taken during the previous twenty-four to thirty-six hours before the attack, as well as the length of time between meals. Make a note of the time you went to bed and got up, together with any special events that occurred. If you can identify triggers you may be able to avoid migraines in the future. But not everyone can: there are so many possibilities and each one of us is different. So try another tack: keep notes of what action you took to deal with each attack – what drugs you took and when, and what other 'aids' you used such as hot/cold packs, sleep or relaxation. This might help you find the best way to deal with your attacks – or, at least, armed with this personal data, you can get your doctor's help in tackling the problem.

Diet

Apart from blood sugar and food triggers, another point worth noting is that a good diet is very important in helping build up the body's defences. If you look upon migraine as a weakness waiting in the wings to get you when you are low, it makes sense to guard against this situation. A good diet also helps your body combat stress, anxiety and depression which are other well-known triggers for migraine. Many members have recommended a low-fat high-fibre diet.

It is very easy to get into a spiral where you are feeling down, so you eat junk food to console yourself or you hardly eat at all because you can't be bothered, and so on. Your body defences get lowered, leaving you prey to infections, stresses, pressures, allergies and other triggers that you would normally be able to cope with. A good diet with plenty of fresh fruit, vegetables, protein and complex carbohydrates is important.

Doctors

Migraine is an illness. As such you have every right to consult a doctor about yours. Even though he or she may not be able to make them go away, enough information is available to help the GP enable you to handle your attacks and maybe even lessen their frequency or the severity of the pain. If your doctor feels it is necessary, he will refer you to a specialist. Help the doctor to help you by going to the surgery armed with as much information as you can about your migraines. No two migraines are identical, but most of us try to forget about them as soon as the attack is over. So record the details of your attack just after you've had one. Read Chapter 10 and you will know exactly how to go about recording the story of your migraine. You can then go and discuss the matter with your doctor like two experts, you being the authority on the pattern of your own migraine and he being the authority on the medical armoury that exists to help you.

Drinks

If you can, keep drinking through an attack so you won't get dehydrated. Different people find different drinks helpful. Tea can be soothing for those not affected by caffeine. Some members report that they like fizzy drinks at this time, such as bitter lemon and coke. Jo Liddell, Director of the Migraine Action Association, has a pet tip for getting rid of an impending attack. At the first hint, drink three glasses of water immediately. This gets the kidneys working hard and in so doing can often obviate an attack.

Drugs

A wide range of drugs are used in migraine treatment, both for individual attacks and for long-term prevention. Many sufferers need only simple analgesics, available over the counter. These include paracetamol, aspirin, ibuprofen or one of the proprietary compounds. Soluble or effervescent tablets are often better than solid ones because they are more quickly absorbed. If sickness is a problem, some special migraine compound tablets contain anti-sickness formulations. If these don't help sufficiently your doctor may prescribe anti-sickness tablets (also called anti-emetics), to be taken separately before taking any painkillers.

Long-term preventative drugs must, of course, be taken under the supervision of your doctor. These include pizotifen, betablockers, calcium-channel blockers and methysergide (see Chapter 11). Long-term drugs may be prescribed for a set period, say six months, after which they are stopped to see if there has been a long-term improvement. Often headaches stay away sufficiently for long-term treatment to be stopped, at least for a while.

Energy

Some members report that their 'early warning' of an attack is a feeling of extra energy or exuberance. Some say they experience a 'high', while others feel tired or lethargic. Some find that they can 'work off' an attack by doing something very energetic at the first hint of a migraine. Try taking a really close interest in this 'high' or 'low'. Does it only precede a real attack as opposed to a false alarm or a minor one? How long before an attack do you experience this mood change? Would it be a good time to take any medicaments? Or can you prepare yourself for an attack in other ways – get someone else to pick up the kids from school. Take a ready-made meal out of the freezer or even nip down to the shops and buy one. Depending upon when the signal comes, you can help yourself by taking the pressure off. Get used to looking out for this kind of signal. Make friends with yourself. Listen to what your body is trying to tell you and take action accordingly.

Fatty food

This can be a trigger for some sufferers. Try and avoid this type of meal if you think it may affect you.

Fear

The fear of having a migraine and of making arrangements in case you have an attack is so common that a word has been invented for it – mellontophobia – by Dr J. N. Blau, Co-director of the City of London Migraine Clinic and Honorary Medical Advisor to the Migraine Action Association. It is taken from the Greek word *mellontas*, which means 'to be forthcoming'. So it is the fear of something forthcoming which ruins the lives of many migraine sufferers. Try not to let it happen to you; better to cancel plans and explain the reason, if necessary, than be forced to live a very restricted life.

Flickering lights/television screens

This is a very common trigger. Avoid flickering lights, flashing sun and flickering television or cinema screens if you can. Have your TV adjusted if necessary. A remote control is useful because it enables you to switch off or change channels immediately if something is bothering you. (See also *Fluorescent lights*.)

Fluorescent lights

These come in two varieties – flickering and non-flickering. Psychologists have recently found that people who suffer from agoraphobia – a fear of open spaces – are particularly susceptible to the adverse effects of conventional fluorescent lights. Fluorescent light appears to increase their heart rate and could contribute to panic attacks in the street.

Evidence also shows that some people who do not suffer from agoraphobia are disturbed by this kind of lighting, which is a major cause of office stress. Doctors believe that fluorescent lighting may cause headaches because the flicker interferes with normal eye movements. The best solution is to reduce the flickering by switching to high-frequency fluorescent lighting or to lights which mimic natural daylight.

There is an alternative. Psychologists from the Medical Research Council's Applied Psychology Unit in Cambridge have developed a red-orange coloured tint which cuts the flicker from fluorescent light by a third. They say that wearing glasses with this tint may prevent headaches in susceptible people. The lenses are made by Cambridge Optical and are sold by opticians.

Gastric stasis

It is not uncommon for migraine sufferers to find that painkillers, even very powerful ones, have no effect once an attack is under way. This is because the stomach 'shuts down' during an attack and very little is absorbed, Doctors call this gastric stasis. The drugs given to treat the condition are metoclopramide (Maxolon) or domperidone which also have anti-sickness properties. They make the stomach empty faster so that the drugs pass into the small intestine and are absorbed more easily.

Goggles

Variable Frequency Photo-Stimulation goggles are a new treatment for migraine attacks, developed at the Hammersmith Hospital in London. The goggles flash patterns of bright lights in the left and right eyes alternately. The light output is adjustable from dim to bright. So far, the results of studies seem to be good for sufferers of both classical and common migraine, and some patients have been helped by them. But research is still in progress. Scientists are looking at changes in the electrical activity of the brain during migraines and the effects of using the goggles.

The goggles are available by mail order from Migra Ltd, St James's House, 108 Hampstead Road, London NW1 2LS. They should be used as soon as possible when a migraine is coming on, either during the visual disturbances or when other warning signs are experienced. They can also be used during the headache itself. They can be very relaxing. People who suffer from epilepsy, especially photosensitive epilepsy, need to consult their doctor before using the goggles.

Holidays

Sufferers often find the beginning of a holiday ruined by headaches. The stress and tension of going away can set off an attack. Try and be well organized in advance, and avoid last minute panics. Also arrange your schedule as best you can so as to avoid, for example, missing meals, and very late or early starts. Talk to your doctor: it may be worth taking a preventative anti-migraine drug for a short while when you know you are particularly vulnerable.

Hormones

Women suffer more frequently than men from migraine, and this is thought to be due to the influence of hormones and the monthly cycle. The Pill can affect the pattern of attacks, or they may start once the woman goes on the Pill. After the menopause, headaches may decline or disappear completely. Some women experience migraines before or during their periods, and sometimes also mid-cycle at ovulation time. Some women suffer migraines particularly badly during their period but have less severe attacks at other times. Keeping notes of your own pattern may help you spot your dangerous times. Often migraine clears up during pregnancy, only to return afterwards. In some cases, where migraine attacks occur only at the start of menstruation or a day or two before, and always on the same day of the cycle, hormone treatment can be successful. This can be prescribed by your doctor. (Chapters 3, 4 and 5 discuss hormones and migraine.)

Hot baths

These can sometimes trigger attacks. Others find relief through relaxing in a warm bath when an attack strikes.

Hot dog headaches

Like Chinese restaurant syndrome, these headaches are caused by nitrates and nitrites which are food additives. Cured meat such as sausages, ham, bacon and salami contain these chemicals, which are used to enhance the colour.

Hot packs

Whereas some people like cold packs during migraine attacks, others find it soothing to have something warm gently resting against the face, head or stomach, or even just to cuddle. A hot water bottle is of course ideal, but make sure it is not too hot. Hand hot temperature is about right.

Hypoglycaemia

This is another word for low blood sugar and the majority of migraine sufferers are thought to have a tendency to this condition. Patients with low blood sugar produce too much insulin – the opposite of diabetes where patients produce too little insulin. Symptoms of over-production of insulin are very similar to those of the prodrome or aura stage in migraine – light-headedness, faintness, palpitations, cold sweat and sometimes double vision.

Since low blood sugar is such a strong contributory factor to migraine attacks it is well worth taking the trouble to understand the technicalities involved. In *The Migraine Guide and Cookbook* Josie Wentworth describes the hypoglycaemic situation very well:

Normally, insulin is secreted at frequent intervals in response to the metabolic demand but that is all, whereas the diabetic's secretion of insulin is scanty and insufficient for the body's needs. The hypoglycaemic, on the other hand, receives a continuous outpouring of insulin.

Blood sugar is the fuel for every cell in the body. But, while the other cells derive nourishment from other sources, the brain is nourished by the glucose in the blood. So, as blood sugar or glucose levels drop, depression and a state of panic or nervous tension and anxiety result. The brain is literally being starved and is panicking in an attempt to keep itself functioning.

Hypoglycaemia cannot be cured or controlled by a miracle drug, but it can be controlled by adherence to a special diet. This places the responsibility for controlling the condition entirely on the patient.

You might think that the answer is to add more sugar to your diet. Unfortunately, eating more sugar only aggravates the problem because ingesting it acts as a direct stimulant to the body to produce more insulin and the hypoglycaemic is back to square one. Coffee, or rather the caffeine contained in it, is one of many stimulants to the adrenal which indirectly, but nevertheless surely, instigates a chain reaction which ends up with the production of more insulin.

The answer is to eat little and often and keep your diet varied and light on sugar.

Ice cream headaches

These are caused by a sudden cooling of the roof of the mouth or throat, or by taking very cold drinks quickly. The immediate cause is a sudden stimulation of one of the nerves in the head. Migraine sufferers are no more prone than others to these headaches. The symptoms are a pain or numb feeling in the head or side of the face, which does not usually last very long. The advice is to eat ice cream or imbibe the cold drinks slowly.

Kelp

Some sufferers have found that taking kelp tablets daily helps. Kelp is a natural source of iodine and is said to assist in the working of the thyroid glands.

Lavender oil

Available over the counter, essential oil of lavender rubbed gently into the temples can soothe and relax and may bring some relief. Rosemary oil is also good.

Migraine clinics

These specialized clinics and neurological departments at some hospitals see migraine patients referred by their doctors. The City of London Migraine Clinic and the Princess Margaret Migraine Clinic, also in London, see patients without appointment in an acute, untreated, normal attack which has started that day. By observing patients during attacks, valuable information can be gained. Much research has been done by these clinics and their work continues to unravel the mysteries of migraine. The work of migraine clinics is explained in Chapter 10.

Nausea

For many sufferers nausea can be as big a problem as the headache itself. If sickness prevents painkillers from being effective, anti-sickness pills may be prescribed to be taken separately at the first sign of an attack. These tablets can also be taken in conjunction with painkillers. Some are available as suppositories which is ideal for those who vomit.

Nitrates and nitrites

These are chemicals added to meat, particularly sausages. They dilate the blood vessels and as such can cause headaches.

Overdose

Sufferers may be tempted to take more than the recommended dose of their tablets, especially when nausea makes them seem ineffective. But any tablets swallowed will be absorbed later on when the gastric function returns to normal. If you take more than one drug, remember that they may contain the same ingredients. Read labels and stick closely to recommended doses. Taking too many painkillers can actually cause headaches.

Painkillers

Many sufferers can cope with their attacks using standard over-the-counter painkillers. Others need extra help, or special migraine drugs available only on prescription.

Paracetamol

This drug is effective for some and has the advantage of being free of gastro-intestinal side-effects. The maximum dose is 4g daily – that is, eight 500mg tablets in twenty-four hours. More than this can be dangerous, causing permanent liver damage.

Pillows

Some members have found that migraine attacks that start in the morning are related to their sleeping posture at night. There are special pillows on the market that ensure correct alignment of the neck while you sleep. But an ordinary soft pillow can be moulded into the required shape.

Relaxation

Learning to unwind can help some sufferers, especially where stress is a trigger. You can learn relaxation techniques by going to classes in your locality. Relaxation for Living has trained teachers who run classes in different parts of the country. They also do correspondence courses and sell books and tapes on relaxation by Jane Madders, who did a great deal of work on teaching relaxation and stress management at migraine clinics and was also one of the founders of Relaxation for Living. More about relaxation appears in Chapter 13.

Research

Much research into migraine is now being carried out all over the world, and modern scanning equipment has made it possible to examine changes in the brain that were previously impossible to detect. At one time there was a division of opinion as to whether migraine was primarily a disorder of the nervous system or of the cardiovascular system (the heart and blood vessels). At the moment the medical profession seems to be focussing on the nervous system and research is concentrating in that area. Members of the Migraine Action Association have helped by raising money, filling in questionnaires giving blood samples and taking part in drug trials.

Sex

Some sufferers have complained of migraine attacks following sexual intercourse. There are two types of headache involved, says the Diamond Headache Clinic. In the first, the excitement accompanying intercourse causes muscle contraction in the head and neck which leads to the headache. The second type is often called an 'orgasmic headache', and this is thought to be caused by an increase in blood pressure which causes the blood vessels to dilate. The amount of physical exertion involved in intercourse does not seem to be relevant. The pain, which usually appears just before or at the moment of orgasm, is usually very intense and centred around the eyes; it can last for a few minutes or several hours.

Of course there is always the blood sugar angle. So try not to indulge on an empty stomach and if it is going to be a marathon event take a break and eat. This can obviate a migraine attack. It is, after all, a question of using up energy so the same rules apply.

Sinuses

If you have sinus problems it is worth trying to get them cleared up for the beneficial effect on your migraines. One patient told us that he had suffered migraines for many years when his doctor suggested that he had an X-ray on his sinuses. They were found to be blocked. The patient underwent a simple operation on his nose and was prescribed a nasal spray for daily use. His migraines, he says, have virtually ceased.

Often patients suffering from migraine are diagnosed and treated for sinusitis. The area affected by sinus headache is usually above the eyes or below the eyes. These areas are usually very tender. Chronic sinus disease very rarely causes head pain. Acute sinusitis, associated with a fever and a blocked sinus, can on the other hand cause headache.

Smoking

Migraine can be triggered or aggravated by smoking, according to the Diamond Headache Clinic. It can cause biological changes in the blood and blood vessels, and this can happen just by being in a smoke-filled room. Smoking can trigger or increase the severity of cluster headaches.

Sports headaches

Some people suffer a migraine after they have played sports. There is an easy answer here. Take one glucose tablet before you play sports and then one straight after, and follow this with a snack like a sandwich a few minutes later – after a shower and a change of clothing.

Stress

Sufferers often quote stress as a major factor in triggering migraine attacks. This is not surprising when you consider that our bodies are not really equipped to handle long periods of stress. Centuries ago when we were hunters the body was tuned to quick action stress: when faced with a threatening situation we either stood our ground and fought, or ran. This-fight-or-flight response has become part of our psychological and physical make-up.

What happens when we prepare for action, says Dr Paul Bebbington in *Handling Stress*, is that the brain receives a warning signal which triggers a chain of reactions throughout the body. Stimulated by an alarm hormone, the adrenal glands secrete adrenalin which mobilizes the body's defences and prepares it to fight or run. The heart pumps more blood and more oxygen to the muscles. Blood vessels in the skin and stomach constrict, enabling more blood to be diverted to the brain. The lungs bring in more oxygen, and as the body temperature rises we start sweating in order to cool down. Then another hormone, cortisol, is released by the adrenal glands to make sources of energy available from other parts of the body to stabilize the situation.

This was all very well for primitive man, but it does not help us cope with the kind of stress we are faced with today. In modern life stress, pressure and anxiety can be with us day in, day out for months and years. So we have to find other ways of coping. Obviously the most efficacious way is to identify the cause of the stress and get rid of some or all of it. That may mean changing your job, or moving house, or cutting down on social activities. It's not easy to reconstruct your life in this way. What's even more difficult, sometimes, is to come to terms with what is causing the stress, because you don't want to give up an activity or let people down. This problem is often best solved with the help of a professional counsellor.

There are, of course, many on-going stressful situations that we cannot do anything about. The thing to do is to make time for yourself and do something that you enjoy regularly. This can be a hobby, sporting activity or anything else that you like, so long as you do it often enough. Meditation, yoga and relaxation techniques are other good ways of helping the body handle stress. More details are given in Chapter 13.

Sunshine

Hot, humid weather and bright sun often bring on migraine in susceptible people. Use dark glasses and a broad-brimmed hat when you are outside. Try to block out flashing sunlight if you are driving – wear sunglasses and a hat, or put the blinds up if you are a passenger. Low winter sun is a particular hazard.

Tartrazine

Also known as E102, this is a yellow food colouring which is thought to trigger migraines in some people. If you think it affects you, note that it is included in the yellow Migraleve tablets.

Tea

The caffeine content of tea may affect some sufferers. If you want to see whether it affects you, try cutting it out for a while and drink decaffeinated tea instead. Conversely, many sufferers find a hot cup of tea relaxing during an attack. If you think caffeine affects you try herbal tea.

Television

Flashing and flickering lights can trigger migraine. A remote control for the television is useful since it enables you to change channels immediately should the one you are watching start to flicker.

Tiger balm

One member has reported that rubbing tiger balm on her forehead and the back of her neck can bring relief during an attack. You can get this ointment from chemists. If applying it on children, don't get it in their eyes as it can sting. Also, anyone strongly affected by smell should probably steer clear of this treatment as it has the kind of sharp smell that is very good for unblocking sinuses!

Travel

Travelling is still a major problem for migraine sufferers. Dehydration seems to be one of the factors and many members have written to the Association to say that they take a lot of liquid with them – not the very sugary kind as a rule – whether travelling by car or aeroplane. One member said she takes a flask of black coffee with her on long journeys and makes herself keep drinking it at regular intervals. She says other liquids will do as long as they don't have milk or sugar in them. Other members find that drinking copious amounts of very diluted squash helps – and, of course, make sure that you have little nutritious snacks with you so that you do not get caught out on the no-food syndrome. It is also worth taking bottled water with you in the car or on aeroplane journeys. You never get enough on charter flights.

Car journeys can be a nightmare for migraine sufferers. A number of factors may combine to cause problems. Glare from the sun, especially if it flashes through the side windows, is difficult to cope with, but you can try wearing sunglasses and a peaked hat. One solution, offered by a member, is to buy a three-inch-wide strip of transparent plastic from a car accessory shop. Cut the strip to the shape of the top edge of the side windows. It adheres like cling film and you can trim it so that the lower edge of the film cuts out the light from the sky but does not obscure the view of side roads. Be very careful not to use a colour which 'kills' the red of the traffic lights as you could misjudge the colour of traffic lights on side roads. Another member suggested that passengers stick a piece of card to the side of their glasses to block out the sun.

Noise on car journeys is another problem and members have suggested that passengers wear ear defenders like those worn by shooters, tractor drivers and chainsaw operators. Ear plugs, particularly mouldable ear plugs, are also useful. It may be worth fitting sound-proofing to your car. Stop for frequent breaks and remember to eat regularly too. Eat something before you set off and don't munch on chocolate bars as you go along. Try to set off early to avoid worries about getting there on time. Again, if you are a passenger it may help to use a neck cushion.

Incidentally, travel sickness pills have helped some migraine sufferers on any type of journey.

Triggers

There are an enormous variety of triggers for migraine sufferers: foods, smells, flickering lights, bright lights, noise, stress, tiredness, change of routine including sleep pattern, changes in the weather, hot baths, excitement and so on. The key is to try and find your own triggers. Keep a note of everything you ate or did during the thirty-six hours preceding each attack. Over several attacks you may be able to spot a common factor. Try to think what was different about the day before the attack. If attacks are only at the weekends, do you get up later? Is the time in between meals longer? If attacks occur only during the week, what do you do at the week-end that is different? Do you eat more? Relax more? Get to know the pattern of your migraine and, if possible, what triggers an attack. In other words: fight back!

Understanding

In addition to understanding as much as you can about your migraines, it is important that friends, family and work colleagues understand the problems too. In the past, migraine sufferers have had to put up with a lack of sympathy from others who thought migraine was just a fancy word for headache. It is not. It is an illness. This book was written so that you, the sufferer, can gain some background information about the condition. But that is only a small part of the story. It has been written by a sufferer for sufferers about sufferers and is backed by the organization that represents us all. By reading the stories of other sufferers, you can see that you are not alone or making a fuss. There are over 6 million migraine sufferers in the UK – some hardly notice their attacks, while others get very ill with them. Most illnesses are like that.

If your friends or family look perplexed when you get a migraine or don't seem to understand why you are so ill during an attack, get them to read some of the true stories in this book. They don't need to read the medical stuff. What matters is that they understand what it feels like to be a sufferer. The pain and sickness are shared by a great many of us – most of us otherwise as able-bodied as the next man or woman, and certainly as sane.

Understanding is a two-way street. Most of us are aware that by being ill so regularly we are putting our families under some strain. But maybe we are not always good at telling them we understand that our migraines give them problems as well. Make a point of telling your family and friends that you know it is rough on them too. Knowing that you know can often be a help.

VDUs

If you use a personal computer or word processor, make sure that the monitor has a rock-steady display and does not flicker or shimmer. Also, a black background with white or green characters seems to give less glare than black on a white background. Arrange the room lighting so that it does not reflect off the screen or the keyboard, or go straight into your eyes. Remember that fluorescent lighting can be a problem, too, as already discussed.

VDU work should be limited to a maximum of four hours in any one working day or 50 per cent of the working time, whichever is the shorter. You should have regular breaks – one hour's work should be followed by a few minutes' break. Incidentally, EC regulations state that VDU users are entitled to have a screen filter fitted to their terminals to cut down glare and reflection and to control static and dust (see Hazel's story in Chapter 6).

If you are about to start using a VDU for the first time it is a good idea to get your eyes tested so that future examinations can reveal any deterioration. You should in any case have your eyes checked regularly if you work on one. The optician may be able to add an anti-glare device to the prescription of your lenses.

Warning signs

Getting to know your own warning signs is probably the first step in a self-help regimen to prevent or curtail the severity of attacks. Here are some of the most common ones, listed alphabetically and not in order of significance:

- Change of bowel function
- Constant yawning
- Depression
- Excitability
- Exhilaration
- Irritability
- Mental aberrations
- 'Phantom smells' which aren't really there
- Pins and needles sensations
- Speech difficulties
- Tension
- Thirst or fluid retention
- Unusual energy
- Unusual hunger
- Unusual pallor
- Unusual tiredness
- Visual disturbances
- Weakness and trembling

Water

Some members recommend drinking plenty of water on a daily basis, and at the first sign of an attack. Drink at least half a pint of water, tepid if you can, if you feel a migraine coming on. This will activate the kidneys and may abort the attack.

Weather

Members have reported that certain kinds of weather seem to trigger attacks. Bright winter sunlight, shining at a low angle, triggers those who are normally triggered by bright and/or flashing lights. Cold winds (see below) can make the face ache and trigger a migraine in some. Nearly everyone, even non-sufferers, can get a headache in humid or thundery weather.

The effects of weather on headache frequency were studied at the Diamond Headache Clinic in Chicago. A rapid fall in atmospheric pressure has, in the past, been cited as a weather trigger for migraine headaches. Other triggers reported include strong winds, hot and cold weather, thunderstorms and seasonal changes. The Clinic studied a hundred migraine patients for twenty-one months. The researchers concluded that weather did not, as a rule, play an important role in migraine, but they felt that some individuals might be more susceptible to rapid extreme changes. They also felt that for some sufferers weather might play an important role in conjunction with other well-known factors such as stress.

Wind

Cold, biting winds can sometimes trigger an attack. So if you are going out in this type of weather, cover your head and as much of your face as you possibly can. Hot, dry winds can also trigger headaches.

X-rays

Migraine does not show in X-rays but many people have X-rays and scans to eliminate any other possible causes of their symptoms.

Yawning

Excessive yawning is often a sign of an impending attack.

Yeast

This substance has been found by some to trigger attacks. It is present, of course, in a great many foods and also in vitamin B tablets. You can find yeast-free versions of the latter in health shops.

Zzzzzz :

Sleep is very important in the treatment of migraine. After an attack, sleep is the best recuperation there is. But sleep is also known to play a part in triggering migraines. Too much sleep is a known offender – this is thought to be due to a drop in blood sugar. Some sufferers find that they wake up with a migraine after a 'lie-in'. This could be because the patient has gone much longer than usual without eating or drinking anything. The solution is not to say in bed for more than an hour longer than usual or, if you do, make sure you have something to eat and drink at your bedside.

Deep sleep is another cause. Alcohol or sleeping tablets can cause you to sleep longer than your body really needs, which can induce a headache. If you find you are going through a phase of sleeping more deeply than usual and are waking up migrainous, try drinking a large glass of water or other non-alcoholic liquid before going to bed. There is nothing quite like a full bladder for hindering sleep!

Too little sleep is also thought to provoke attacks, but not quite so much is known about this. Sleeping less than your body needs will of course lead to tiredness, which leaves you prone and vulnerable to all sorts of illnesses, including migraine. Stress may be at the bottom of it, and learning to relax may help (see Relaxation). If you are a bad sleeper you may find that meditation techniques help (see Chapter 13) and you may like to try the 'sleep' cassettes and literature produced by Relaxation for Living (see Relaxation).

Useful Addresses

The British Acupuncture Council
Park House, 206-208 Latimer Road
London W10 6RE
0181-964-0277

The Society of Teachers of the Alexander Technique
20 London House, 266 Fulham Road, London SW10 9EL

The Amarant Trust
Sycamore House, 5 Sycamore Street, London EC1Y O5R
0891 660 620

International Society of Professional Aromatherapists
82 Ashby Road, Hinckley, Leicestershire LE10 1SN

Aromatherapy Organisations Councils
P.O. Bo 355, Croydon CR9 2QP
0181-251-7912

Register of Traditional Chinese Medicine – see The British
Acupuncture Council

The Sino European Clinics Ltd
Manvers Chambers, Manvers Street, Bath BA1 1PE
01225-483393

The British Chiropractic Association
Equity House
29 Whitley Street, Reading, Berkshire RG2 0EG
0118-950-5950

The British Homoeopathic Association
27a Devonshire Street, London W1N 1RJ
0171-935-2163

The following homoeopathic hospitals or clinics treat patients on the National Health Service:

Bristol Homoeopathic Hospital
Cotham, Bristol, Avon BS6 6JU
0117 973 123

Glasgow Homoeopathic Hospital
1000 Great Western Road, Glasgow G12 0YN
0141 211 1600

Mossley Hill Hospital
Park Avenue, Liverpool, Merseyside L18 8BU
0151 250 3000

Royal London Homoeopathic Hospital
Great Ormond Street, London WC1N 3HR
0171-837-8833

The National College of Hypnosis and Psychotherapy
12 Cross Street, Nelson, Lancashire BB9 7EV

British Migraine Association – See Migraine Action Association

The General Council and Register of Osteopaths
56 London Street, reading, Berkshire RG1 4AQ
0118 957 6585

The British School of Reflexology
92 Sheering Road, Old Harlow, Essex CM17 0JW
01279 429 060

Migraine Action Association (previously British Migraine Association)
178a High Road, Byfleet, West Byfleet, Surrey KT14 7ED
01932 352-468

Relatation for Living
Distress Management Training Institute
Foxhills, 30 Victoria Avenue, Shanklin, Isle of Wight PO37 6LS
01983 868166

Transcendental Meditation
Freepost, London SW1P 4YY
0800 269 303 (free of charge) or

Freepost WN510 37R
Skelmersidale, Lancs WN8 6BR
0990-143-733

The British Wheel of Yoga
1 Hamilton Place, Boston Road, Sleaford, Lincs NG34 7ES
01529 303 233

Bibliography

Advice from the Diamond Headache Clinic: Seymour Diamond, MD and Judi Diamond-Falk, International Universities Press, Inc New York

The British Medical Association Guide to Medicine and Drugs: Dorling Kindersley

Handling Stress: Paul Bebbington, Mental Health Foundation

Migraine: Oliver Sacks, Faber and Faber

Migraine: Clinical, Therapeutic, Conceptual and Research Aspects: edited by J. N. Blau, Chapman and Hall

Migraine – The Facts: F. Clifford Rose and M. Gawel, Oxford University Press

The Migraine Guide and Cookbook: Josie A. Wentworth, Corgi

Migraine and Headaches: Marcia Wilkinson, Martin Dunitz

Migraine Special Diet Cookbook: Cecilia Norman, Thorsons

Once a Month: Katharina Dalton, Fontana (an imprint of Harper Collins)

Relax – And Be Happy: Jane Madders, Unwin Paperback

Stress and Relaxation: Jane Madders, Macdonald

Understanding Headaches and Migraines: Dr J. N. Blau, Consumers Association and Hodder and Stoughton

Acknowledgements

I should like to thank Jo Liddell, director of the British Migraine Association, for her help and support while I was writing this book and to Dr Anne MacGregor, M.B.B.S., of the City of London Migraine Clinic for her invaluable help in checking the manuscript for medical accuracy. My thanks also to Geoffrey Robinson, O.B.E., for his assistance. But most of all I am deeply indebted to the many migraine patients who told me their stories so openly. Although most of the names have been changed their stories are true and I believe that their generosity of spirit will bring comfort to migraineurs all over the world.

Jenny Lewis November 1992

Index

To order your copies from Vermilion (p&p free) telephone TBS DIRECT on: 01206 255 800.

Gut Reaction
by Gudrun Jonsson

'I've got a very good gut feeling about Gudrun and her work.'
Terence Stamp

Most of us accept that diet has a profound effect on our overall health and well-being. Gudrun Jonsson believes that the best diet in the world counts for nothing if you don't digest your food properly. *Gut Reaction* explains how malabsorbed foods build up in the digestive system as toxins, undermining our vitality, our immunity to disease and ultimately our health. *Gut Reaction* shows how you can reduce this toxicity by following a unique regime combining sound nutritional advice, homeopathy and reflexology. The results are startling and include:
* steady weight loss
* increased levels of energy
* a boosted immune system
* a reduction of most allergy-induced illness
* clarity of mind

Direct, simple, empowering and proven for people of all ages, follow *Gut Reaction* and aim for health, energy and happiness.

Price: £7.99
ISBN: 0 09 181673 4

The Power of Positive Thinking
by Norman Vincent Peale

This book could change your life.

Norman Vincent Peale's international bestseller, *The Power of Positive Thinking* has inspired millions with his heartfelt prescription for enjoying a more fulfilling life.

The Power of Positive Thinking is a simple, practical, heartfelt guide to enable everyone to enjoy confidence, success and joy. Norman Vincent Peale, the father of positive thinking and one of the most widely read inspirational writers of all time, shares his famous formula of faith and optimism which millions of people have taken as their own simple and effective philosophy of living. His gentle guidance helps to eliminate defeatist attitudes, to know the power you possess and to make the best of your life.

Price: £7.99
ISBN: 0 7493 0715 3

No More PMS!
by Maryon Stewart with contributions from Dr Alan Stewart

The original top-selling guide advocating a medically proven, positive and wholly-natural approach for treating your PMS problems.

No more PMS. No more suffering. Success in under four months.

This practical guide is the 5th edition of *Beat PMS Through Diet*. It has been fully revised to include personal success stories and the results of ground-breaking research from the Women's Nutritional Advisory Service programme. Drawing on over fourteen years of success in treating PMS, Maryon Stewart explains how to evaluate your symptoms and how to devise a tailor-made diet which could cure your own PMS problems. She includes the latest advice on:
* how to make essential dietary changes;
* the role of nutritional supplements;
* the importance of magnesium;
* taking moderate exercise on a regular basis.

There really is no longer any need to suffer with PMS.

Price: £8.99
ISBN: 0 09 181622 X

More Books from Vermilion
The prices given were correct at the time of going to press